Validity Issues in Quantitative Migrant Health Research

Challenges in Public Health

Editor: Prof. Dr. Oliver Razum, Bielefeld

Formerly/früher: Medizin in Entwicklungsländern
Herausgegeben von
Prof. Dr. Hans Jochen Diesfeld, Heidelberg

Band 58

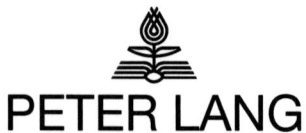

PETER LANG

Frankfurt am Main · Berlin · Bern · Bruxelles · New York · Oxford · Wien

Patrick Brzoska
Oliver Razum

Validity Issues in Quantitative Migrant Health Research

The Example of Illness Perceptions

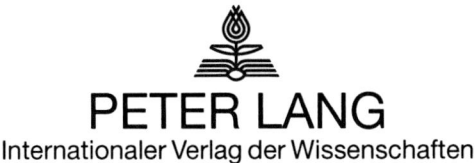

PETER LANG
Internationaler Verlag der Wissenschaften

Bibliographic Information published by the Deutsche Nationalbibliothek
The Deutsche Nationalbibliothek lists this publication in the Deutsche Nationalbibliografie; detailed bibliographic data is available in the internet at http://dnb.d-nb.de.

The printing of this publication was supported by a grant from the European Union (DG SANCO) as part of the MIGHEALTHNET project.

ISSN 1863-768X
ISBN 978-3-631-59448-3

© Peter Lang GmbH
Internationaler Verlag der Wissenschaften
Frankfurt am Main 2010
All rights reserved.

www.peterlang.de

Table of contents

Figures

Tables

Abbreviations

AIDS	Acquired immunodeficiency syndrome
CASI	Computer-assisted self-interview
CFA	Confirmatory factor analysis
CHA-CA	Chance/accident attributions
CSQ	Consequences (scale)
CVD	Cardiovascular diseases
EFA	Exploratory factor analysis
ERP	Emotional representations (scale)
F-SozU K-14	Short Social Support Questionnaire/Kurzform des Fragebogens zur sozialen Unterstützung
HBM	Health Belief Model
HIV	Human immunodeficiency virus
HRQOL	Health-related quality of life
IAQ	Interviewer-administered questionnaire
ILC	Illness Coherence (scale)
IMM-CA	Immune attributions
IPQ	Illness Perception Questionnaire
IPQ-R	Revised Illness Perception Questionnaire
IQOLA	International Quality of Life Assessment Group
KMO	Kaiser-Meyer-Olkin (coefficient)
MAP	Minimum average partial test
MCS	Mental composite score/scale
MeSH	Medical subject headings
MI	Myocardial infarction
MSA	Measure of sample adequacy
NA	Negative Affect
PA	Positive Affect
PANAS	Positive and Negative Affect Schedule
PCA	Principal component analysis
PCR	Personal control (scale)
PCS	Physical composite score/scale
PSY-CA	Psychological attributions
RF-CA	Risk factor attributions
SAQ	Self-administered questionnaire
SF-36, -12, -8	The Medical Outcome Short Form Health Survey 36, 12, 8
SHG	Self-help group
SPHS	Self-perceived health status
SRM	self-regulatory model

SVR	Sachverständigenrat zur Begutachtung der Entwicklung im Gesundheitswesen, Advisory Council on the Assessment of Developments in the Health Care System
SWE	General Perceived Self-Efficacy Scale/Skala zur Allgemeinen Selbstwirksamkeitserwartung
TCR	Treatment control (scale)
TLA	Timeline acute/chronic (scale)
TLC	Timeline cyclical (scale)
TPB	Theory of Planned Behavior
TRA	Theory of Reasoned Action
US	United States (of America)
WHO	World Health Organization
ZfT	Zentrum für Türkeistudien/Center for Studies on Turkey

1. Why culture matters in quantitative health research

Migrants and ethnic minorities compose an increasingly large proportion of the population of Germany and other European countries (Razum et al. 2008; Boswell 2005). In order to study the health of these population groups as well as possible health disparities, professionals and researchers are faced with the challenge to apply multicultural and multi-language adaptations of research instruments (Porter/Gamoran 2002; Ercikan 2002; Harkness 1998). Of particular importance are psychometric instruments, i.e. instruments aiming to measure psychological constructs, such as health-related quality of life or well-being. However, although these constructs, response behavior and language usage may differ between populations of different cultural and ethnic background (van de Vijver 2001; American Psychological Association 2003; Padilla 2001), possible methodical problems emerging from this divergence are often neglected. Quantitative research, for example in epidemiology, is often based on the questionable assumption that cultures are homogenous and that instruments are transferable across different population groups (Hunt/Bhopal 2004). A famous example is the International Pilot Study on Schizophrenia started by the World Health Organization in the late 1960s (WHO 1973). It aimed to identify and compare diagnostic patterns, prevalences and clinical courses of schizophrenia in different parts of the world. Yet, cultural aspects had neither been taken into account in the survey process nor in the analysis phase of the study, resulting in highly controversial findings (Haasen et al. 2005). While in many disciplines similar issues have been discussed for decades, health research seems to be reluctant to tackle this topic. This is highly problematic, since health-related research often deals with constructs that are inherent to culture, thus putting the results obtained by the respective studies in question. When it comes to research involving migrants and/or ethnic minorities, additional challenges come into play that, currently, hardly any discipline sufficiently accounts for. One of the fields where many of the shortcomings mentioned above are particularly obvious is the evolving research on illness perceptions.

Illness perceptions are an important component of illness self-regulation and thus are also relevant for coping with illness (Leventhal et al. 1992; Leventhal et al. 1992; Hampson 1997). Their consideration, therefore, should be regarded as crucial for adequate health care provision (Petrie/Weinman 1997; Hagger/Orbell 2003; Myers 2003; Rothman et al. 2003). This is particularly important for migrants and ethnic minorities (Becker 1984; Adler et al. 1996; Hampson 1997; Petrie et al. 2003). The Illness Perception Questionnaire (IPQ) (Weinman et al. 1996) and its revision (IPQ-R; Moss-Morris et al. 2002) proved to be valuable instruments for the assessment of illness perceptions. Their validity and reliability have been empirically tested and they were successfully adapted for a number of different diseases and applied to different research questions. Also, a short version of the IPQ-R, the Brief IPQ, is available allowing a more rapid assessment of illness perceptions and the application to a wider range of population groups. Both the long and short form of the instrument would also be useful for culturally sensitive care of Turkish migrants in western European countries such as Germany. However, although a Turkish version of the IPQ-R, validated in Turks residing in Turkey, exists, its psychometric properties have never been assessed for Turkish migrants residing in Germany. Of the Brief IPQ, no versions validated in either foreign languages or cultures are available.

This book contributes to filling this gap. It assesses the psychometric properties of the IPQ-R and the Brief IPQ in Turkish migrants residing in Germany, with the latter instrument being translated as part of this venture. By doing so—and by using the assessment of illness perceptions as a case study—this is one of the few publications illustrating the methodical challenges of applying mainstream quantitative instruments to migrants.

Chapter 2 describes the role of validation and cultural adaptation and deals with the use of instruments in migrant health research. Chapter 3 provides an introduction into the theory and measurement of illness perceptions. It highlights the role of illness perceptions from a cultural perspective and tells about the public health relevance of considering illness perceptions in health care provision. Furthermore, the revised and the brief version of the Illness Perception Questionnaire are described in detail. Chapter 4 is dedicated to the case study on the examination of illness perceptions in Turkish migrants. It outlines its methodical aspects and illustrates its findings. Also, this chapter assesses the quality of the adapted instruments by comparing their properties to the validity and reliability of the original versions. In chapter 5, we draw conclusions regarding the requirements for a full-scale validation of the IPQ-R/Brief IPQ in Turkish migrants. Based on this example, we discuss additional challenges involved in research aiming to make quantitative comparisons across cultures.

2. Application of instruments in quantitative health research

A crucial step in every empirical study is to apply instruments that allow an accurate assessment of the topic in question. In new research fields or for research questions dealing with constructs, concepts, or risk factors that have never been studied before, researchers need to develop suitable instruments first, usually starting by exploring the research field and applying qualitative methods. Results and experiences gained here form the basis for the development of quantitative instruments and the generation of hypotheses. This development usually travels through a set of different phases in which the research problem is defined, the instrument drafted on the basis of prior knowledge, its items analyzed and selected, and finally revised and validated. In many cases, however, researchers analyze specific questions in research fields where already much knowledge is available. Here, they can draw on instruments developed by others and pursue their research interest directly. A combination of both becomes relevant when instruments well tested and validated for one population need to be applied to another population. If this population differs in language and/or culture, adaptation for either one or both becomes necessary. For two reasons, this is an issue of increasing importance. First, in psychology, social, and health sciences, oral and written self-report measures are highly relevant. In times of shared decision making, much of planning in health care systems is based on this form of data collection (Hanna et al. 2008). Second, due to growing diversity and international migration, researchers are increasingly faced with barriers to collecting self-reported information in migrant population and/or ethnic minorities since these groups often have little competency in the language of the target country. Also, psychological constructs might be different between different cultural groups (American Psychological Association 2003; Padilla 2001). Hence, instruments that examine constructs well in one population are not necessarily applicable to other populations without adaptation. This is where validation comes into play. Validation is the process of assessing the validity and other quality criteria of an instrument (see chapter 2.2). Only if instruments prove sufficient quality in a population they were properly adapted for, they can be used in this population for the assessment of relevant variables.

2.1 Current practice in migrant health research

The relevance of cultural adaptations has been discussed in sociology for many decades. However, knowledge and practical experiences gained here are not sufficiently adopted in quantitative health research. For example, as regards epidemiology, Hunt/Bhopal (2004) criticize that many language translations and adaptations are inadequate, ignoring divergence in psychological constructs and response behavior, and often using a level of language not appropriate for most individuals of minority groups due to low education. In order to avoid hassles related to adapting instruments properly, epidemiological and clinical studies in many cases exclude ethnic minorities, especially when individuals are not proficient in the language of the majority population. This, however, leads to non-representative findings (Bartlett et al. 2003). In other cases, cultural hegemony and transferability of concepts is taken for granted where caution would be advisable. For instance, for research on health-related quality of life (HRQOL) in the US, Stewart/Napoles-Springer (2000) showed that many studies on non-English speaking persons use translations not appropriate to the constructs assessed by the original version, ignoring the need for adaptation in order to account for cultural diversity. Another issue concerns the comprehensibility and properties of instruments and their application to patients of the same language in different countries. In this case, it is known that the validity and reliability of these instruments may differ. Hence, of the major instruments (e.g. the Short Form Health Survey 36, SF-36) different versions of the same language exist for different countries (e.g. Spanish for Spain, Argentina, Costa Rica, and the US or English for the US, Taiwan, New Zealand, and the Philippines). How important such versions are can be easily demonstrated by comparing the semantic difference of the same language in different countries (see also chapter 5.2.1). For example, the Spanish verb *coger* means *to take* in Spain while it is used derogatively for *having sex* in Mexiko. Similarly, *guagua* means *baby* or *child* in Peru and Colombia while it means *bus* in the Carribean (cf. Spielberg et al. 2005). Differences in languages can also be observed for "younger" migrant groups like Turkish migrants residing in Germany (Hinnenkamp 2002; Backus 2006). In cultural research on health, this needs particular attention, because words to describe states and traits may differ across different (sub-)cultures (Anastasi 1972).

These "migrant versions", however, are only available for very few instruments and for a limited number of languages. Where no such versions exist, it is common practice in quantitative migrant health research to use the translated and validated instrument versions of the respective native populations without prior testing of the instruments in the migrant target populations (cf. for instance Koochek et al. 2007 who apply the Farsi version of the SF-36 in Iranian migrants residing in Sweden). This is also true for research on Turkish migrants in Germany (cf. for instance Akbiyik et al. 2008 who apply the Turkish version of the Beck's Depression Inventory, Tagay et al. 2008 who apply the Turkish version of the Hospital Anxiety and Depression Scale, and Nickel et al. 2006 who apply the Turkish version of the State-Trait Anger Expression Inventory in Turkish migrants residing in Germany without prior validation). In these and many other cases, the good performance of instruments in these populations is implicitly taken for granted and possible validity problems, among other things due to differences in socio-demographic background, language, and culture as compared to the source population, are not discussed. This is highly problematic, since it is known that Turkish migrants residing in Germany are not representative for the Turkish population of Turkey. Most of first-generation Turkish migrants originally came from rural Eastern Anatolian sites, holding conservative values, little school education, and little proficiency in reading and writing (Şen/Goldberg 1994). Naturally, instruments validated and considered good in the native population highly likely behave differently when administered to Turkish migrants. Most of the literature on this subject usually does not cover this problem. Although this migrated population's language and cultural background resemble the language and cultural background of the country of origin, adaptation for both could be necessary, since both are influenced by the process of migration (Mangalam 1968; Kerswill 1994). Especially, the effect of migration on language has only little representation in literature on psychological testing and assessment.

2.2 Test criteria of psychometric instruments

It is not in the scope of this book to give an overview of the theories, concepts, characteristics, and the construction of psychometric instruments. However, dealing with validation, one is bound to at least outline basic criteria that allow determining the quality of psychometric instruments. "Psychometric" refers to the measurement of psychological concepts and constructs, such as knowledge, stress, HRQOL, attitudes, or, as in the present case, illness perceptions. According to Stevens (1946), measurement can be defined as "the assignment of numerals to objects or events according to rules" (ibid, p. 677). The tools of measurement in psychology are test instruments and very often questionnaires. Different criteria exist informing about the quality of a psychometric instrument. Following Lienert (1989), they can be categorized into primary and secondary criteria (Fig. 1). The latter include

- *test efficiency* that exists when instruments allow a fast assessment, are applicable as group instruments, and are easy to apply and to analyze;

- *test fairness* that tells whether different person groups, e.g. of different age, sex, and religion, have the same chances of reaching comparable results in the test;

- *test utility* that exists when an instrument allows measurement, description, or prediction of a concept or construct that has high relevance in research and practice and for which no suitable instrument existed before;

- *test comparability* that exists when similar instruments gain comparable results as the instrument in question;

- *test reasonableness* that tells about the degree of mental, physical, and time-related test-taker burden (ibid, Bühner 2006).

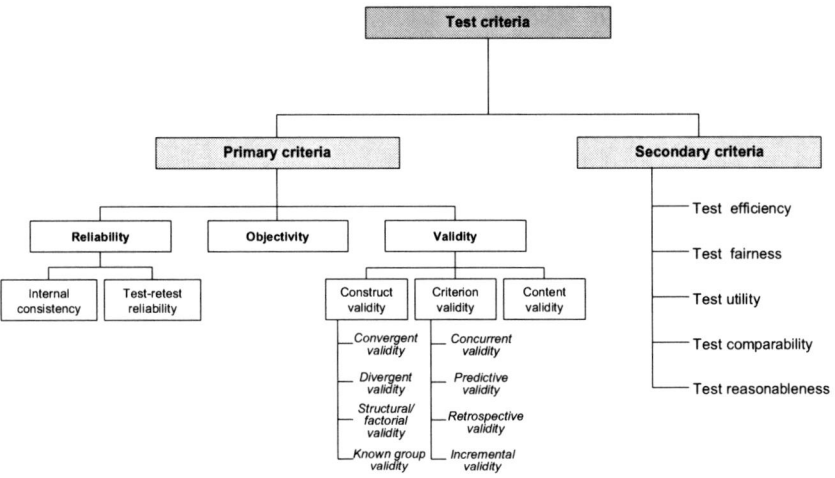

Fig. 1: Quality criteria for psychometric instruments
(Source: Own illustration based on references cited in chapter 2.2)

However, more important than these aspects are primary criteria comprising reliability, objectivity, and validity.

Reliability

Reliability tells about the repeatability and consistency of a measurement. An instrument is considered reliable if it is independent from unsystematic measurement errors that influence test results at random. Reliability comprises the two criteria "internal consistency" and "test-retest reliability". The former is usually considered in questionnaires, when multiple item scales are applied that are all supposed to measure the same variable. *Internal consistency* (most frequently measured by Cronbach's α) then refers to the correlation between the items of a scale and describes the degree to which each item measures the same higher-order variable. *Test-retest reliability* is measured by administering the instrument to the same group of people at two different time points (t_0 and t_1). Thus, it is a measure of stability over time. The correlation of results gained at t_0 and t_1 represents the repeatability of results, with higher values (according to a rule of thumb these should be at least >0.7) indicating a better quality of the instrument (Kline 2000; Bühner 2006; Hinton 2004).

Objectivity

Objectivity refers to the degree to which results gained by an instrument are independent from the researcher in terms of procedure, analysis and interpretation (Bühner 2006).

Validity

Going back to Latin *validus* or French *valide* (meaning "strong" or "powerful"), validity in the context of psychometric instruments can be defined as the extent to which an instrument measures what it was designed for to measure (Bryant 2000). There are different types of validity that can be further subdivided (ibid).

Most important is the *construct validity* of an instrument, a term sometimes used synonymously with validity in general. In a more narrow sense, however, construct validity comprises convergent validity and divergent validity. An instrument has high convergent validity when it gains results comparable to other well-tested instruments in the field that measure the same or very similar concepts. These already existing instruments may even be the gold standard in examining a particular construct but may have severe drawbacks such as high test-taker burden which motivate researchers to develop new instruments. While for the assessment of convergent validity similar instruments are correlated, divergent validity is assessed by correlating instruments measuring different constructs. Here, conversely, low correlation coefficients are desirable, because instruments should be construct-specific, i.e. not measuring more than one construct. "Known group validity" refers to the ability of an instrument to discriminate between distinct subgroups of a population who have different characteristics. "Structural" or "factorial"" validity usually refers to the validity of the instrument's factor structure, most frequently assessed by factor analysis. Known group and factorial validity are sometimes considered a third and fourth sub-type of construct validity (Kline 2000).

Criterion validity (also labeled "concrete validity") describes to what extent an instrument measuring latent constructs is related to concrete real-world outcomes. It can be divided into four different subtypes. Concurrent validity tells how well an instrument correlates with other criteria assessed at the same time. An example is the correlation of a test of concentration and results in a school exam. Predictive validity refers to correlations with criteria that are assessed in the future, like the correlation between intelligence and final grade point average or the correlation of illness beliefs and disease outcomes. Retrospective validity, conversely, refers to the relationship of current results and criteria assessed in the past (e.g. intelligence scores assessed in graduate students and their correlation with school grades) (Bühner 2006). Incremental validity, usually determined by hierarchical regression models, tells about the degree to which an instrument adds to the predictive power of other instruments (Hunsley/Meyer 2003).

Unlike construct and criterion validity, *content validity* (also known as "logical validity") is not determined by means of coefficients, but is based on content related considerations (Kline 2000; Bühner 2006; however, Lashwe 1975 proposed a quantitative approach to its measurement based on qualitative experts' opinions). Content validity refers to the degree to which an instrument represents all aspects of a given construct. Thus, based on theoretical knowledge it can be argued that the revised version of the IPQ has a higher content validity than the original version since it represents the SRM construct of Leventhal more comprehensively (e.g. by also assessing emotional representations, something that the original version did not offer; see chapter 3.2).

While test-retest reliability and predictive validity are assessed using a follow-up design, the other validity sub-groups usually are assessed by means of a cross-sectional approach. However, these validity types, in addition, can also be assessed longitudinally. For example, longitudinal convergent validity refers to the ability of an instrument to correlate with other instrument over time (Liang 2000).

This categorization of types of validity must not be confused with the terms "internal" and "external" validity. While the types of validity described above are elements of the Classical Test Theory and tell something about the quality of instruments, internal and external validity tell something about the quality of a study design. *Internal validity* concerns the accuracy of findings and asks whether the study design is appropriate to generate accurate results and to reveal characteristics of the subject in question. *External validity* refers to the generalizability of findings to populations, settings, and times other than those studied. This concerns, among other things, the sample's quality and representativity for its statistical population, as well as the choice of inclusion and exclusion criteria.

2.3 Migration and health

2.3.1 Migrant groups residing in Germany

Within the past several hundred years, persons with a migration background have become an important part of German society. With 15.4 million people today, they represent almost one fifth of the German population (Statistisches Bundesamt 2009). Germany's migrant population consists of 7.3 million people without German citizenship (foreign nationals) and about 8.1 million people with migration background holding a German citizenship. The latter comprise Germans of whom at least one parent is a foreigner or an *(Spät-)Aussiedler*, i.e. a re-settler of ethnic German origin usually from Eastern Europe. With a population of 1.9 million, Turks are the largest foreign nationals group in Germany. Additionally, some Turks have adopted German citizenship (0.5 million) and others have received German citizenship at birth (so far, no numbers are published about the size of this group). These three groups make people of Turkish background (in the following referred to as "Turkish migrants") the second largest ethnic minority in Germany. However, much of the data that is available in health reporting only refers to Turkish nationals.

2.3.2 Migration, social inequalities and illness

Migration commonly refers to the movement of people either within a state ("internal migration") or across national borders ("international migration") (cf. Bryjak/Soroka 1997). Especially, the latter is often a process that initiates a cascade of critical life events, representing an intergenerational break in the biography as well as the personal and social development. In general, migrants are exposed to different health-related challenges that distinguish them from the population of the target country (Razum et al. 2004; Geiger/Razum 2006). These challenges, however, are not the result of epidemiological factors alone. To a large extent, they also go back to the interaction of living conditions, values, traditions, culture, and social factors in the country of origin and the situation in the target country.

For the case of international migration in developed countries, the health situation and health access of migrants, in the long run, is worse than that of the majority population (Dias et al. 2008; Claassen et al. 2005). This also applies to the migrants in Germany (Razum et al. 2008; Machleidt et al. 2007; Brucks et al. 2003) and has several reasons. Although migrants can in part rely on particular resources such as strong social support through close family bonds and "mutual obligation" (White 1997, p. 757), their overall social and economic situation is worse than that of Germans. Examples are higher rates of unemployment and poverty, lower income, lower education, and disadvantageous living conditions (Razum et al. 2008). Due to this situation, their overall access to health care is limited which is further facilitated by diverging cultural beliefs, tradition, language barriers, and social discrimination. However, challenges migrants are facing go far beyond the situation they are exposed to in the target country and are the result of influences they experience through their entire life course. To take this perspective into account, Spallek/Razum (2008) present a model that highlights different risk factors migrants are exposed to at different points in their lifetime. These start with factors related to heredity, pass over to factors related to the living conditions and the social environment in the country of origin and the changes involved in the process of migration (e.g. loss of social contacts and strain caused by acculturation pressure), and finally to factors determined by the situation in the target country. All these risk factors contribute to the differences between migrants and the native population of the target country with regard to health and health care needs, finally resulting in health inequalities. As a consequence, the health situation of migrants is worse than that of Germans. Although representative data on migrant health in Germany is missing, research indicates that the disease pattern of migrants and Germans is different. A study from Hamburg, Germany shows that foreign nationals residing in Germany as compared to Germans have higher rates of age-associated illnesses and a higher prevalence of mental disorders (Freie und Hansestadt Hamburg 1998; see Razum et al. 2008 for an overview about further results). Longitudinal analyses of the German Socio-economic Panel (*Sozio-oekonomisches Panel*, SOEP) further indicate that foreigners have a worse self-perceived health status as compared to indigenous Germans (Zeeb et al. 2005; however, see Ronellenfitsch/Razum 2004 for contrasting results about migrants from Eastern Europe). As the migrant population that today has a younger age structure than non-migrant Germans gets older, also their prevalence of age-associated diseases will increase. Estimates show that the proportion of foreigners aged 60 or older on all foreigners will more than double by the year 2030 (Münz/Ulrich 2001). Hence, also their probability of contracting chronic diseases will increase, making cultural sensitive health care services for migrants more important than ever.

2.3.3 Culture, ethnicity, religion, and coping with illness

Aside from social factors, cultural background has a substantial impact on health and illness behavior, especially when it greatly differs from the cultural mainstream of the target country. Most of the Turkish migrants are Muslims and religion plays an important role for them, as a study by the Bertelsmann Foundation has highlighted (Thielmann 2008). Consequently, cultural and religious aspects require strong consideration in the health care process and may differ even more from the majority population than they do in other migrant groups in Germany with a Christian background, such as Ethnic Germans of Russian origin (*Russlanddeutsche*, Russian Germans) (Brzoska/Razum 2009).

Culture is a multidimensional construct referring to tradition, language, customs, art, and science of a society. It is a set of mutually defined rules allowing the cultivation of social relationships and interpersonal communication, acquired by individuals as part of their socialization. Culture "serves" different purposes. It creates a collective identity that ties individuals to society and that passes down social characteristics to subsequent generations (Trotter 1988). Culture is related to *ethnicity* that, however, is a broader construct of which culture can be considered just one part. Ethnicity refers to a group of people with similar culture, characteristics, beliefs, traditions, and identity. This similarity distinguishes one ethnic group from the other and contributes to mutual segregation. In order to define one's own ethnic membership, individuals participate in dynamic processes in which they exclude others from their own identity by denying characteristics in others they attribute to themselves and by attributing characteristics to others claiming to be non-existent in their own group (Weber 1978; Cohen 1978). In literature, however, the term "culture" is usually used for reasons of familiarity, referring to a general system of beliefs and values and forming the identity of a population group. This usage will also be adopted in this thesis. A third construct relevant in the context of disease coping and migration is *religion*. Although there is no clear definition of what religion is, it can—for the purpose of practicability—be defined as a set of symbolic systems, traditions, and cultural phenomena related to some kind of supernatural power and influencing behavior (King 2005). Sometimes, also the construct of *spirituality* is used instead of religion because it is not restricted to supernatural beliefs, but considers the self-concept of a person (Greenstreet 2006a; Meraviglia 1999). However, in many cases it is used interchangeably, especially in health sciences (Emblen 1992). Culture and religion together form a particular identity and value systems of a cultural group.

Spallek/Razum (2008) describe how different factors contribute to health differences in migrants throughout lifetime. Although not explicitly stated by the authors, also the influence of culture and religion should be considered in a life course perspective, especially in a migration context. By means of migration, individuals with a particular culture developed against the backdrop of a particular situation in the country of origin clash with a cultural environment in the target country that is structured differently. This foreign and to a certain degree incompatible environment is perhaps not able to sufficiently address norms and value systems these migrated populations hold. Hence, it is also likely that diverging health concepts, health care needs, and health behavior—all influenced by culture—are not adequately approached by the health care system.

The influence of culture on health and health behavior results from psychological and social factors. Among other things, culture has an impact on the perception of pain, gender, reproduction, diet, anatomy, stress, and the patient-provider relationship (Helman 2000). Furthermore, it influences the way people experience, interpret, and cope with illness and how they behave in illness therapies (e.g. Chia et al. 2006). Similar associations have been found for religion (e.g. Greenstreet 2006b; Pargament et al. 2001; Ano/Vasconcelles 2005). As will be shown in chapter 3.4, individual explanatory frameworks for diseases and disease development highly differ with culture. As for patients with a Turkish background, experiences from clinical practice show that these patients have a holistic view of their body, their health, and their illness. Following the argumentation of Berg (2001), this holism can create conflicts in the German health care system that tends to separate body and soul from each other. This conflict arising from culture-specific needs of migrants on the one hand and the culture of the target country not being able to address these needs properly on the other hand bears possible problems. Although standard care services start to take the particular needs of migrants into account aiming to reduce the gap between culture-specific needs and current clinical practice, health care for migrants is still suboptimal (e.g. Wunn 2006; Weilandt/Altenhofen 1997; Spallek/Razum 2007). This might in part be responsible for suboptimal coping strategies in migrants that have frequently been mentioned in German literature. For instance, they become evident when we look at the field of motivation to therapy where minority groups, as compared to the majority population, have considerably low rates of adherence

(Gosciniak 1997; Eberding/von Schlippe 2000; Ozankan 2008). The same phenomenon was reported for minorities in other countries (Chia et al. 2006; Lip et al. 2002). Therefore, effective intervention strategies for ethnic minorities have to consider this diversity in order to provide proper support for disease management. For this purpose, knowledge about the characteristics of coping with illness in migrants is necessary because it allows adjusting current therapies and services to their particular needs and helps to improve their coping strategies. Several national and international studies (e.g. Becker 1984; Adler et al. 1996; Hampson 1997; Petrie et al. 2003) have proposed differing illness perceptions as being one of the most crucial reasons for problems in disease coping among ethnic minorities. They are an important element in the "self-regulation" of illness and differ strongly between different cultural groups.

•

3. Illness perceptions and the self-regulatory model

3.1 The theory of self-regulation in chronic illness

One of the main purposes of health psychology is to explain, predict, and influence health related behavior of individuals, including the choice of coping strategies, such as adherence to therapies and participation in rehabilitation programs. In the past, different psychological models of health behavior have been developed serving this purpose. In the course of this development, models have become increasingly sophisticated. While early models concentrated on isolated factors, newer models and theories represent multicausal and multidimensional systematic frameworks (Glanz et al. 2002). Especially, social-cognitive models have gained popularity in research on health behavior and health behavior change. Of these, the Health Belief Model (HBM) is the most popular one. It is still widely applied today. Since it also forms the basis for more complex models, it will be briefly outlined in the following.

According to the HBM, different core factors influence the health behavior of individuals (Fig. 2). Most important are the components of perceived severity of and susceptibility to disease that form the overall threat an individual perceives over his or her illness. The perceived threat is appraised against the backdrop of benefits (decreasing the risk for a severe disease) and costs (uncomfortability, strain, pain, necessary resources) of the behavior itself. Furthermore, the individual takes into account his or her ability to perform a particular behavior (self-efficacy as known from the social-cognitive theory). Finally, the individual considers internal and external cues to action (e.g. incentives to perform the behavior, reminders, media publicity or information on how to perform the behavior). Depending on how these four core components are evaluated against one another, the respective behavior is either carried out or not (Janz et al. 2002).

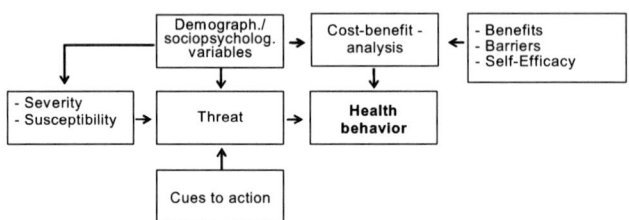

Fig. 2: The Health Belief Model (Source: Own illustration following Janz et al. 2002)

The predictive power of the HBM can be enhanced by combining it with elements of newer social-cognitive models, of which most important are the Theory of Planned Behavior (TPB) and its sub-model, the Theory of Reasoned Action (TRA). The TPB and TRA complement the HBM approach by adding the component of outcome expectation and normative beliefs about social expectations (Montaño/Kasprzyk 2002). Although these models can predict intention to behavior change rather than behavior change itself, they are widely used in research on coping behavior, e.g. research on adherence (Christensen 2004).

In terms of their practical value for the explanation of cultural differences in patterns of chronic disease coping, it can be criticized that social-cognitive models do not sufficiently cover the self-concept of a person, neglecting that health to a substantial extent is a subjective construction. Especially, when it comes to coping with illness, perceptions of health and illness can be crucial, but lack adequate representation in social-cognitive models.

Both in English and German language literature, there is a profound discussion about the construction of health and illness. However, both scientific communities approach this topic differently. While in the case of the former mostly quantitative methods are applied today, German researchers dealing with that subject usually choose a qualitative approach. Also, concepts and definitions of underlying constructs differ. The German author Faltermaier talks about "subjective health perceptions" (*subjektive Gesundheitsvorstellungen*) which he defines as ideas, beliefs, and considerations relevant to health. These perceptions comprise "subjective health and illness theories" *(subjektive Gesundheits- und Krankheitstheorien)* and "subjective health concepts" *(subjektive Gesundheitskonzepte)* (Faltermaier et al. 1998; Faltermaier/Kühnlein 2000; Faltermaier 2002). English language literature, however, does not subordinate perceptions of illness to subjective health perceptions. Instead, terminology refers to the topic as "perceptions of health and illness" in general. Although different expression for "perceptions of illness" exist here, too (e.g. illness beliefs, illness representations, illness schemata, and illness cognitions), they are used interchangeably in almost all cases. This usage will also be adopted in this book. Also, by focusing on two quantitative instruments, this report follows the research tradition from English language countries and approaches illness perceptions by means of quantitative methods (see Filipp/Aymanns 1997 and Faltermaier 2005 for a further outline of different research traditions). Although a qualitative approach applying an exploratory framework makes it possible to examine illness perceptions very thoroughly, it is limited to a small number of individuals. Quantitative research, however, enables researchers to examine illness beliefs on the level of the general population which facilitates the implementation of this examination into clinical practice more easily.

According to Heider (1958), laymen behave like scientists who try to find explanations for events occurring in their daily life. In this context, Heider coined the expression of "causal attribution", describing that individuals attribute particular causes to certain events. These attributions indirectly affect their behavior. The onset of a chronic illness usually is such an event nurturing the desire for some kind of explanation which persons usually respond to with their illness representations. In literature, illness representations have been mainly conceptualized using the self-regulatory model of illness (SRM) developed by Howard Leventhal and colleagues (Leventhal et al. 2001; Diefenbach/Leventhal 1996; Hampson 1997; Leventhal et al. 1980; Leventhal et al. 1992). It has proved to be a valuable framework in the examination of patients' illness representations of different diseases and in different cultures (Hagger/Orbell 2003). The SRM considers health and illness behavior as being driven by previous experiences and subjective theories of illness. These theories originate from a dynamic decision making process and go far beyond the representations of causal attributions of illness and the components of severity and susceptibility that are conceptualized as the core dimensions of health behavior in the HBM. Horne (1997) succinctly summarizes this SRM concept in five questions around which patient behavior is clustered when it comes to illness: "[W]hen people think about illnesses they appear to organize their thoughts around five key questions: What is it? (Identity). How long will it last? (Timeline). What caused it? (Cause). How will it/has it affected me? (Consequences). Can it be controlled or cured? (Cure/Control)" (ibid, p. 157). Patients develop representations as a result of the answers they find to these questions. These representations then form the basis for coping strategies dynamically chosen in the course of illness (Fig. 3).

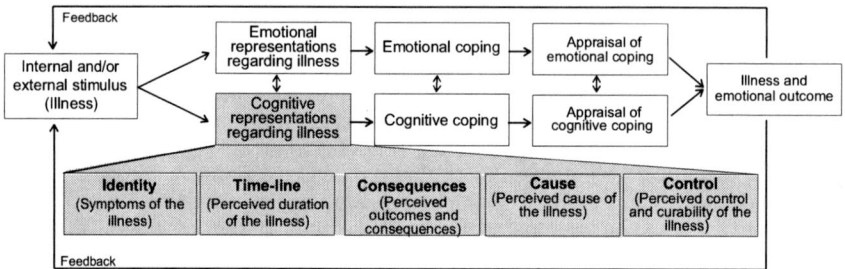

Fig. 3: The self-regulatory model according to Leventhal (Hagger/Orbell 2003, p. 144; Leventhal et al. 2003, p. 50; modified)

The SRM conceptualizes patients as active problem solvers who try to harmonize beliefs, coping strategies, and the appraisal of these strategies. By doing so, illness perceptions affect the choice of coping strategies, have an effect on the patient's outcome expectation and finally on the outcome itself. Illness perceptions, coping strategies, and disease outcomes are related to one another, with coping strategies moderating the relationship between illness perceptions and disease outcome. As already mentioned, coping strategies are chosen dynamically and are based on experiences gained throughout the course of life. They are modified or replaced when considered non-effective or non-compatible with previous experiences. Because of this appraisal process, the self-regulatory model is also known as the Common Sense Model because, for the individual, coping strategies, illness representation, and disease outcome have to be consistent among each other. Consequently, it would not be enough to only consider objective criteria in the evaluation of patients' coping strategies. By neglecting the role of experiences, coping strategies being suboptimal from an objective point of view usually cannot be understood by professionals who are not aware of the subjective context of the patients although these strategies could make sense when reflected in light of previous experiences patients have gained. These experiences are responsible for the phenomenon that coping strategies regarded as the optimal response to a given condition by professionals sometimes do not make any sense for patients. This can be easily illustrated using the example of antihypertensive therapy: Patients undergoing this therapy are often confronted with the confusing situation of having to take medication against a condition that does not cause any symptoms. Instead, the therapy sometimes makes them feel worse because of floppiness and drowsiness due to blood pressure decrease. For them, not taking this medication instead of following the prescribed regimen is the common-sense reaction to their condition. This results in the coping strategy of non-adherence—potentially dangerous, but creating a meaning ("making sense") for the patient. Considering this example, it becomes pretty clear that it is more likely that patients choose an optimal coping strategy when their knowledge, perceptions, and experiences are compatible with the therapeutic regimen and the symptoms experienced.

Apart from the five core dimensions, the illustration in Fig. 3 shows the two stage process character of the SRM comprising cognitive and emotional beliefs, developed simultaneously following a stimulus such as the onset of a disease. This two stage process character, for instance, takes the possibility into account that perceived consequences of a disease can lead to fear that, as an emotional representation, can have an effect on coping behavior and can result in a strategy which is problem-based and focused on emotion (Moss-Morris et al. 2002).

Lay beliefs of illness are related to beliefs about medicines concerning perceived adverse or long-term effects of medication taking. Beliefs about costs and benefits of medication can result in positive or negative effects on coping procedures. Also, beliefs and expectations about the therapeutic regimen itself are relevant and depend on the knowledge and the quality of the patient-provider relationship (Horne et al. 1999; Horne/Weinman 1999; Horne 1999). Beliefs about medicine and therapy can also be conceptualized over Leventhal's SRM and are subject to an entire branch of research on self-regulation. Therefore, they cannot be covered here in greater detail. However, illness perceptions, beliefs about medicine and about therapy together form a triad of therapy/disease related cognitions that, through a subjective cost-benefit-analysis, constitute a dynamic system in which all components of self-regulation are interrelated and permanently adjusted to one another in a feedback loop.

3.2 Quantitative measurement of illness perceptions

Since illness perceptions are not influenced by culture alone, but rather are a result of environmental factors interacting with personal factors, it is not possible to assess representations theory-based on the level of entire cultural groups. Instead, this assessment has to be incorporated as part of assessing needs on an individual level.

While there is agreement in literature over the five relevant core dimensions of illness representations, different instruments for assessing these dimensions have been proposed. Apart from open-ended and semi-structured qualitative approaches, different quantitative instruments have been applied in the past decades of which only few have practical relevance today. Due to lack of suitable instruments, quantitative studies on illness beliefs used to be restricted to the assessment of one or two dimensions simultaneously. Examples of instruments used for that purpose are the Survey of Pain Attitudes, the Pain Beliefs and Perceptions Inventory, the Beliefs about Pain Control Questionnaire, the Schema Assessment Instrument, the Respiratory Illness

Inventory, the West Haven-Yale Multidimensional Pain Inventory, and the Health Locus of Control Scales (Scharloo/Kaptain 1997). The Implicit Models of Illness Questionnaire by Turk et al. (1986) was the first instrument that allowed a thorough examination of illness belief dimensions. It defines illness perceptions over four dimensions comprising seriousness, personal responsibility, controllability, and changeability. However, in current research, most of these instruments have little or no representation as a literature search reveals (see Appendix B for the search method applied). Only the Health Locus of Control Scales (Wallston/Wallston 1982) and the West Haven-Yale Multidimensional Pain Inventory (Kerns et al. 1985) are still applied today more frequently, despite being limited to only one or two aspects of illness perceptions.

The Illness Perception Questionnaire (IPQ)

Until the development of the Illness Perception Questionnaire by John Weinman and colleagues (Weinman et al. 1996) in 1995/96, quantitative studies due to lack of suitable instruments never examined illness representation on a thorough basis simultaneously assessing the five core dimensions outlined above. The Illness Perception Questionnaire (IPQ) proved to be a valuable instrument in serving this purpose and today (in its revised form, see below) can be considered the gold-standard in quantitative research on illness perceptions. Using this instrument, it is possible to easily assess illness perceptions utilizing the well-tested self-regulatory framework of Leventhal, while simultaneously compensating shortcomings of older quantitative instruments used in this field. The IPQ is a general, i.e. disease non-specific, instrument theoretically derived from the SRM. The original version published in 1996 (ibid) comprises five scales with 38 items, allowing statements about the five cognitive dimensions of the SRM.

The field of *identity* comprises twelve common symptoms (e.g. "pains", "nausea", "headache", "loss of strength") whose frequency respondents are asked to rate on a four-point scale ranging from "4=all the time" to "1=never". For the purpose of analysis, item values are summed-up, with higher scores representing higher number of symptoms. Representations of *timeline* (3 items, e.g. "My illness will last for a long time"), *causal attributions* (10 items, e.g. "Diet played a major role in causing my illness"), *control* (6 items, e.g. "There is a lot I can do to control my symptoms"), and *consequences* (7 items, e.g. "My illness has had a major consequence on my life") are rated on a five-point response scale from "5=strongly agree" to "1=strongly disagree", some items being inverted. Analysis for the fields of timeline, consequences, and control is done by calculating the respective mean score, with higher scores representing stronger representations. Items in the field of causal attribution are analyzed separately or, depending on the research field and research question, clustered into categories.

The IPQ has been validated in 848 patients from nine different disease groups (hospitalized myocardial infarction (MI) patients, n=143; discharged myocardial infarction patients after 3 months, n=104; discharged myocardial infarction patients after 6 months, n=91; patients with chronic fatigue symptoms, n=115; patients with rheumatoid arthritis, n=22; patients with type 2 diabetes mellitus, n=88; patients with chronic pain, n=60; patients suffering from renal disease, n=32; and patients with asthma, n=193). Internal consistencies (only provided for the MI sample) for the identity, timeline, consequences, and control dimension were satisfactory ranging from Cronbach's α=0.73 to 0.82. The instrument showed a good test-retest reliability in the renal sample (Pearson r=0.68 for control and consequences, r=0.84 for identity, and r=0.49 for timeline) as expected for a stable condition like renal disease. In contrast, test-retest reliability after 3 and 6 months was low for the sample of MI patients indicating, for an unstable condition such as MI, a dynamic character of lay beliefs as conceptualized by the SRM. Convergent, divergent, and predictive validity were also satisfactory. For the latter, the control and the consequences dimension was negatively correlated with the perceived likelihood of future MI.

The Revised Illness Perception Questionnaire (IPQ-R)

In 2002, Jane Moss-Morris and colleagues (Moss-Morris et al. 2002) published a revised version of the IPQ (IPQ-R) in which the timeline and control scale had been improved. The revised version of the instrument (see Appendix C.1) subdivides the dimension of timeline into acute/chronic (e.g. "My illness will last a short time") and cyclic (e.g. "My symptoms come and go in cycles"). The field of control is subdivided into "personal control" and "treatment control". Additionally, new scales were introduced focusing on coherence and emotional representations—two core dimensions of the SRM which are not properly represented in the original version. The respective scales consist of 6 items (e.g. "I have a clear picture or understanding of my illness" with higher values pointing at stronger coherence and "I get depressed when I think about my illness" with higher scores pointing at higher emotional representations, respectively). Except for the addition of new items, the revised version of the IPQ is quite similar to the original with regard to its response format and general appearance. The only substantial change concerns the implementation of the identity dimension. Unlike in the original version, symptoms are not rated by intensity anymore. Instead, patients are asked using yes-no questions whether they have experienced a particular symptom since the onset of their disease and whether they think that this symptom is related to their disease.

Based on its layout and response format, the IPQ-R can be divided into three parts: Part I assessing illness identity by means of 14 items with a double yes-no format, part II examining beliefs about controllability, timeline, emotional representation, and consequences by means of 38 items with a 5-point Likert scale, and part III applying the same response format and presenting 18 items on causal attributions and an additional open-ended item asking respondents to list three causes they think are most relevant for the origin of their disease.

As with the IPQ, validity and reliability of the IPQ-R have been empirically tested (ibid). The IPQ-R validation study slightly differed from that of Weinman et al. (1996). In total, 711 patient were recruited who came from eight different illness groups (asthma, n=86, type 2 diabetes, n=73; rheumatoid arthritis, n=76; chronic pain, n=63; acute pain, n=35; MI, n=47; multiple sclerosis, n=170; HIV, n=161). Principal component analysis (PCA) of the 38 items of the second part of the IPQ-R revealed 7 factors as outlined above. In the third part consisting of 18 items, 4 factors were identified (psychological attribution, risk factors, immunity, and accident or chance). All dimensions showed good internal consistencies (Cronbach's α ranged from 0.79 for cyclical timeline and 0.89 for acute/chronic timeline). As conceptualized by the SRM, the symptoms experienced and the identity subscale showed significant differences indicating that illness identity differs from somatization. The IPQ-R performed well regarding test-retest reliability, as examined on the renal sample after 3 and 6 weeks, with all but one dimension ranging above r=0.5. Satisfactory results were also found for divergent, known group, and predictive validity. They will be described in comparison to the results of the current study in the discussion section of this report.

Adaptability of both the IPQ (for studies published prior to 2002) and IPQ-R (for studies published from 2002 onwards) has been proven for a variety of different illnesses. This includes, for instance, diabetes (Paschalides et al. 2004; Searle et al. 2007), cardiac diseases (e.g. Petrie et al. 1996, Cooper et al. 1999, Petrie et al. 2002), Morbus Addison (Heijmans 1999), Morbus Huntington (Helder et al. 2002), breast cancer (Buick 1997), chronic obstructive pulmonary disease (Scharloo et al. 2000), chronic fatigue syndrome (Moss-Morris et al. 2003), HIV (Gauchet et al. 2007), migraine (Lanteri-Minet 2007), and mental conditions (Lobban et al. 2005a/b; Fortune et al. 2004). Furthermore, the instrument has been used in research on perceptions of infertility (Benyamini 2008).

The Brief Illness Perception Questionnaire (Brief IPQ)

In 2006, a short 9-item version of the IPQ, the Brief IPQ, was published and showed good reliability and validity (Broadbent et al. 2006). It uses a single item approach to assess illness beliefs on an 11-point linear scale (see Appendix C.2). The rationale of the scale development was to develop questions that best fit the content of each IPQ-R subscale. This way, cognitive representations are represented by 5 items (consequences, timeline, personal control, treatment control, and identity; items 1-5), emotional representations by 2 items (concern and emotions; items 6 and 8), and illness comprehensibility by 1 item (item 7). The ninth item assesses causal attributions by an open-ended item format asking patients to rate the three most important causes of their disease. This item is also a part of the IPQ-R causal items. By means of this format, the Brief IPQ allows a rapid assessment of illness perceptions and the application to an even wider range of population groups, repeated-measure designs, and large studies where illness perceptions are only part of a larger set of psychological variables. Seven studies used the Brief IPQ in the past, as listed in the major databases up to October 2009 (see Appendix B for search methods).

The instrument was validated in patients of six illness groups (n=891): MI (n=103); renal disease (n=132); type 2 diabetes (n=119); asthma (n=309); minor illnesses comprising allergies, colds, and headaches (n=166), as well as chest pain (n=62) and showed overall good psychometric properties. Test-retest reliability (measured in the renal sample) was slightly higher than for the IPQ-R with only the comprehensibility item after 3 weeks and the personal control item after 6 weeks showing correlation coefficients r<0.5. Convergent validity, as measured by means of the correlation of the Brief IPQ scales to the full version, is described as being sufficiently high. However, while all other dimensions show correlations of r≥0.5, correlations of the two control scales are only r=0.3. The Brief IPQ proved to predict different outcomes following MI, e.g. participation in rehabilitation, return to work, anxiety, and quality of life, and is able to discriminate between different diseases well.

Translations of the IPQ-R and the Brief IPQ into different languages

The IPQ has been translated into different languages, e.g. German (Franz et al. 2007), Spanish (different translations: e.g. Marcos et al. 2007 for a sample of eating disordered patients and Vázquez et al. 2005 for a sample of hypertensive patients), Tongan (Barnes et al. 2004), Greek (Anagnostopoulos/Spanea 2005), Italian (Giardini et al. 2007), and Turkish (Kocaman et al. 2007; as most of the other language versions online available from http://www.uib.no/ipq/). However, it has been used without published validation for instance by Franz et al. (2007), Anagnostopoulos/Spanea (2005), and Barnes et al. (2004) for different research questions. Besides, the instruments were often adapted for the specific needs of the research question (e.g. psychiatric condition in the study by Franz et al. 2007) and remained unpublished. Only Giardini et al. (2007) and Kocaman et al. (2007) did actual validation studies for the Italian and Turkish version, respectively, without changing the underlying structure of the instrument. Both research groups applied an exploratory framework using exploratory factor analysis for validation although a hypothesis-testing approach (e.g. by using confirmatory factor analysis) would have been more appropriate (Bühner 2006). The Italian version has been validated in 277 inpatients from Montescano hospital from seven different disease groups (hospitalized MI patients, n=70; coronary artery by-pass graft surgery, n=52; chronic heart failure, n=47; valve replacement, n=20; obstructive sleep apnea syndrome associated to obesity, n=53; and respiratory failure, n=35). It showed good psychometric properties and validity and the same factor structure as the original version. The Turkish version was validated in 337 patients with physical illness admitted to Istanbul University hospital and also showed properties similar to the original version. Both versions will be described in chapter 4.3 in greater detail. Validations were also conducted by Marcos et al. (2007) and Vázquez et al. (2005). However, in the course of validation, the instruments were modified and the seven factor structure of the IPQ-R was changed.

Although different translations of the Brief IPQ into foreign languages exist, none of them have been formally adapted or validated.[1]

---

1   After the empirical part of this case study had been completed, a Turkish translation of the Brief IPQ (translated by Serap Batmaz Oflaz) appeared on the internet on a website dedicated to the Illness Perception Questionnaire (http://www.uib.no/ipq/). This website was down since 2005 and was re-launched mid-2008, among other things with new content regarding different translations of the IPQs. Hence, the Turkish translation of the Brief IPQ as translated by Oflaz could not be considered. Instead, an independent translation of the Brief IPQ was created in the preliminary phase of this study. Olfaz' translation, however, will be discussed and compared to the current translation in chapter 4.3.

3.3 The role of illness perceptions for coping behavior

Different studies highlight the role of illness perceptions for different aspects of coping behavior and illness outcomes. Two examples, the role of illness beliefs for attendance at rehabilitation programs and for adherence to long-term cardiovascular therapies, will be presented in the following by means of a short literature review and complemented by a brief overview about other relevant outcomes.

Attendance at rehabilitation programs

Already prior to the development of the IPQ authors have suggested that illness perceptions can affect and predict patient participation in rehabilitation programs. They assumed that programs can only be successful when illness perceptions of patients are compatible with the characteristics of the therapy. They further assumed that intervening into these perceptions can improve adherence and disease outcomes (e.g. see Petrie/Weinman 1997). Although literature is not consistent on that point, the majority of studies supports this assumption. A literature review (see Appendix B for methodical aspects) shows that in total there are ten studies dealing with that subject.

Petrie et al. (1996) examined illness beliefs of MI patients of which one group (n=89) participated in rehabilitation programs and another (n=39) refused participation. Controlling for age and health status, they showed that attendees as compared to non-attendees had stronger beliefs about the controllability ($g=0.40$)[2] and consequences ($g=0.34$) of their disease, the latter only being marginally significant ($p=0.07$). The results, supported by a qualitative analysis of MacInnes (2005), could be replicated by Cooper et al. (1999) in a quantitative study on 137 hospital patients, where attendees had stronger beliefs about the controllability of their disease ($g=0.45$) and stronger beliefs that their own behavior is responsible for their diseases ($g=0.63$). Whitmarsh et al. (2003), however, found contradicting results. In their study on 93 MI patients shortly before the beginning of a rehabilitation program, only higher illness identity and perceived consequences were associated with attendance at rehabilitation ($g=0.77$ and $g=0.67$). Yohannes et al. (2007) examined factors associated with the drop-out of a six-weeks rehabilitation program after MI and found out that weaker beliefs about consequences ($g=0.70$), treatment controllability ($g=0.37$), the perception that the disease is chronic ($g=0.40$), a weaker identity ($g=-0.40$), and a stronger belief about personal controllability ($g=0.46$) were associated with program discontinuation. However, only consequences and controllability remained significant when analysis was controlled for other variables such as age and sex. In a small sample of 62 patients, Petrie et al. (2002) found differences in all categories of the original IPQ, ranging from $g=0.4$ to 0.7 with the contradicting result that lower identity and the perception of fewer consequences were associated with program attendance. These, however, were not significant, which may be due to the small sample size (42+20). French et al. (2005), Petrie et al. (2005), and two theses papers from the University of Brighton, England (James 1999; Cooper 2004) did not find any associations be-

---

2   Hedge's g is used as a measure of effect size. See Appendix B for formulas and an explanation of this concept. If not mentioned otherwise, all reported g's are significant at $p<0.05$.

tween attendance at rehabilitation programs and illness perceptions (see Tab. A 1 in Appendix A for study designs and a general overview).

French et al. (2006) meta-analyzed the studies on rehabilitation attendance published prior to 2006 and found weak but significant associations (presented by point-biserial correlation coefficients, r_{pb}) with illness beliefs (r_{pb}=0.12 for identity, r_{pb}=0.11 for controllability, r_{pb}=0.08 for consequences, r_{pb}=-0.16 for coherence). The authors do not present combined results for causal attributions, because there is no consistent assessment of equal categories between studies. However, three studies assess beliefs about 'stress' and 'own' behavior. Their combined effects show values of $\bar{g}$ =0.24 (CI 0.04, 0.45) and $\bar{g}$ =0.38 (CI 0.18, 0.59), respectively (own calculation), indicating that patients who attribute stress or own behavior to their disease have a higher probability of attending rehabilitation sessions. Confidence levels, though, are quite large what is due to the small number of studies in this combined calculation.[3]

Long term therapies

Some studies have also been done for long term therapies, e.g. after cardiovascular events. Senior et al. (2004) and Ross et al. (2004) surveyed 336 patients with familial hypercholesterinaemia and hypertension, respectively, regarding the adherence to medication intake. They found a significant association between adherence and perceived consequences. Unlike in the studies by Petrie et al. (1996), Cooper et al. (1999), Whitmarsh et al. (2003), and Yohannes et al. (2007), non-adherence was correlated with stronger beliefs about consequences. Furthermore, as Yohannes et al. (2007), Ross et al. (2004) show that perceived treatment controllability is associated with adherence, while perceived personal control is associated with non-adherence. This effect only becomes evident when personal and treatment control are assessed separately, whereas it is missed with instruments that do not distinguish between both concepts, like the original IPQ. This instrument bias may also be the reason why Patel/Tylor (2002) and Senior et al. (2004), each using self-made instruments, found contradicting results. For the very narrow field of adherence to cardiovascular treatment, only Senior et al. (2004) found an association between causal attributions and adherence (g=0.34 for heredity and g=0.17 for cholesterol). See Tab. A 2 in Appendix A for study designs and a general overview.

Byrne et al. (2005) examined the role of illness beliefs for other aspects of health behavior in a large sample of 1611 patients with established chronic heart disease recruited from 35 general practices in Ireland. They found out that patients with higher illness coherence, personal and treatment control perceptions, and lower emotional representations show higher physical activity. However, only emotional representations remained significant in a multivariate model.

Evidence on other aspects

Tab. 1 summarizes the results of a meta-analysis by Hagger/Orbell (2003) that gives a comprehensive overview of associations of the SRM core dimensions with different outcome measures. It becomes evident that these dimensions are associated with almost all the outcomes and that "consequences" and "identity" correlate quite strongly (up to $r_c = -0.67$) with different outcome measures, adjusted for sampling and measurement error. Coefficients are quite robust as can be seen in the high fail safe N (N_{Fs}) that gives the number of studies needed to reduce a coefficient to a non-significant result.

Outcome	Consequences				Control				Identity				Timeline			
	k	N	r_c	N_{Fs}	k	N	r_c	N_{Fs}	k	N	r_c	N_{Fs}	k	N	r_c	N_{Fs}
Physical functioning	15	1849	-.18	39	15	1846	-.03	-	11	1529	-0.28	51	-0.10	1493	-0.10	-
Psychological distress	20	2821	.50	180	20	2817	-.17	48	13	2279	0.36	81	0.20	2182	0.20	42
Psychological well-being	16	2566	-.46	131	16	2566	.21	51	11	2051	-0.37	70	-0.08	2114	-0.08	-
Role functioning	9	1304	-.43	68	9	1301	.04	-	8	1136	-0.56	82	-0.11	1077	-0.11	8
Social functioning	11	1468	-.49	97	11	1465	.13	18	10	1400	-0.48	86	-0.15	1240	-0.15	18
Vitality	6	1171	-.45	48	6	1171	.24	23	6	1171	-0.67	74	-0.18	1171	-0.18	16
Disease state	4	457	-.06	-	4	457	-.17	10	4	457	0.08	-	-0.03	457	-0.03	-

Note. k=number of studies; N=sample size available for each coefficient, r_c=corrected cumulative correlation coefficient; N_{Fs}=Fail safe N. All r_c are significant at $p<0.05$ for $N_{Fs} \geq 0$

Tab. 1: Results of a meta-analysis for the association of SRM illness perceptions dimensions with different disease outcomes (Source: Hagger/Orbell 2003, p. 173)

Similarly, Hagger/Orbell present a meta-analysis of studies highlighting the correlation of SRM dimensions on further aspects of coping behaviors. Less support for an influence of illness beliefs becomes evident for the aspects listed. Unlike for illness outcomes, correlations are rather weak and range from 0.12 to 0.27. However, results are also robust as indicated by high N_{Fs}.

Outcome	Consequences				Control				Identity				Timeline			
	k	N	r_c	N_{Fs}	k	N	r_c	N_{Fs}	k	N	r_c	N_{Fs}	k	N	r_c	N_{Fs}
Avoidance/denial	16	1858	0.23	58	16	1858	-0.04	-	14	1750	0.23	50	16	1858	0.12	22
Cognitive reappraisal	12	1545	0.03	-	12	1545	0.20	36	10	1437	0.03	-	11	1312	0.14	20
Expressing emotions	14	1706	0.21	45	14	1706	0.12	-	12	1598	0.23	43	14	1806	0.02	-
General problem focused coping	15	1800	0.02	-	15	1800	0.27	66	13	1692	0.03	-	15	1800	0.03	-
Specific problem focused coping	13	4765	0.01	-	15	3355	0.12	21	10	2457	0.01	-	9	2359	0.01	-
Doctor's visits	5	1949	-0.01	-	3	1747	-0.02	-	5	1946	0.05	-	4	1888	-0.01	-
Seeking social support	13	1213	0.05	-	13	1213	0.08	8	11	1105	0.05	-	13	1213	-0.04	-

Note. k=number of studies; N=sample size available for each coefficient, r_c=corrected cumulative correlation coefficient; N_{Fs}=Fail safe N. All r_c are significant at $p<0.05$ for $N_{Fs} \geq 0$

Tab. 2: Results of a meta-analysis for the association of SRM illness perceptions dimensions with different aspects of coping with illness (Source: Hagger/Orbell 2003, p. 173)

---

3   Of course, a base of just three studies is rather small for the calculation of summary measures. However, this restriction is not uncommon in literature (see, for instance, Mullen et al. 1992).

Furthermore, Petrie et al. (1996) showed that patients convinced of long-term conse-quences of their disease needed longer for recovery and were longer absent from work than patients with less intense beliefs about consequences. Similar results were found by Lewin (1999) and Weinman et al. (2000). Walsh et al. (2004) found out that illness beliefs are correlated with the time patients take to seek medical care after an acute MI event. Besides, illness beliefs are associated with the degree of continuity of care, i.e. the management of disease over time (Riley et al. 2007).

Considering and targeting illness perceptions in clinical practice

Results from literature suggest that disease outcomes and coping strategies can be improved by changing illness perceptions of patients with the help of intervention programs utilizing the SRM framework. This research question has in particular been focused by Petrie et al. (2002). In a randomized clinical study on patients after MI, they tested a brief tailored hospital intervention aiming at changing patients' illness perceptions against usual care provided by rehabilitation nurses. The short interven-tion comprised three sessions that addressed the SRM dimensions and in which ill-ness beliefs were discussed with patients. The intervention was able to alter patients' perceptions and influenced outcomes positively: Patients in the intervention group as compared to the control group were better prepared for leaving the hospital, returned to work faster, and reported lower rates of angina pectoris 3 months post-MI. Petrie et al. (2002) explain this finding by the dynamic relation of illness beliefs and coping strategies. Because of the feedback loop in which the components of emotional and cognitive representations are permanently adjusted to one another, altering one component affects the entire self-regulation process. Considering this, interventions into this feedback loop by means of tailored programs can be very powerful.

Corresponding illness beliefs between patients and their health professionals have been shown in literature to be crucial for optimal disease management and disease coping. Divergence affects coping and recovery from illness negatively (Mur-phy/Kinmonth 1995; Foulks et al. 1986; Kleinman 1980). Also, as was shown by German authors in early studies, knowledge about patients' illness perceptions is essential to built up an effective patient-provider relationship that is required for posi-tive therapeutic outcomes (Amann/Wipplinger 1998; Becker 1984; Verres 1986). Aside from illness perceptions of patients, Hirani/Newman (2005) stress the impor-tance of illness beliefs hold by patients' families, since differences between families' and patients' illness representations have similar consequences as diverging beliefs on the patient-provider level (e.g. see the studies by Figueras/Weinman 2003 and Kärner 2004).

Due to their role, assessment of lay beliefs should be considered an important part of building a culturally competent patient-provider relationship. The role of discrepan-cies in the patient's and provider's view of illness as an important factor associated with suboptimal coping strategies and poor disease outcomes is especially large in ethnic minorities (see below). It can be assumed that individuals from different cul-tural backgrounds, especially when coming from non-Western societies, highly differ in their representations of illness as compared to Western European societies.

Hence, implementing this assessment is a substantial element of the medical profession and a crucial element of culturally sensitive care.

3.4 Studies focusing on illness perceptions in ethnic minorities

Apart from studies on illness perceptions in different illness groups and for different health behaviors as outlined in chapter 3.3, a huge body of literature exists that examines the role of culture and/or migration on illness perceptions. Most of it uses rather woolly theoretical frameworks to conceptualize illness beliefs and mainly focuses on causal beliefs and beliefs about controllability. This literature reveals huge differences between cultural groups, thus calling for the consideration of illness perceptions in culturally sensitive care. For reasons of brevity, it is not possible to present an overview of the overwhelming amount of studies that highlight differences in illness beliefs in different cultures. Instead, an important paper presenting causal attributions and control beliefs of different cultures world wide will be presented first, before available results on illness perceptions in people of Turkish origin will be outlined.

Causal attributions—Taxonomy and historical considerations

While reports on patient illness beliefs can be traced back to the 16th century, the first systematic studies on illness perceptions in different cultures did not emerge until the last century (Clements 1932). Very famous for its comprehensibility is an ethnographical study on illness beliefs by Murdock et al. (1978), who collected information on causal attributions and control beliefs of 139 cultures from South-, Latin-, and Native North America, East Asia, Sub-Saharan Africa, the Mediterranean region, and from the Pacific Islands. Their study is based on the analysis of ethnographic literature and highlights major patterns of causal and control beliefs in different societies. According to Murdoch et al.'s findings, causal attribution can be categorized into the two groups of natural and supernatural attributions.

Natural causal attributions are based on modern medical science and, for instance, comprise the belief that emotional and physical stress can affect health negatively. Another type of natural beliefs regarded as causing illness is a decline in body function or organic deterioration that, however, could only be found for a few of the examined cultures. The authors state that "in any event, it would seem as though most of mankind considers itself potentially immortal and is unable to conceive of the infirmities of old or middle age in terms other than through the intervention of some hostile agency or force" (ibid, p. 452). Also, accidents play a minor role and are often linked to supernatural causes. Human aggression, finally, considered in many cases to be determined by supernatural powers, bridges the gap to supernatural causes.

The authors identified a far more significant role of supernatural causal attributions which they clustered into the sub-categories of mystical, magical, and animistic causal attributions. *Mystical attributions* comprise the following causes: a) "fate" was found in 28 cultures most of which were complex, b) "ominous sensations" (e.g. looking at the shadow of one's own or dreaming of a recently deceased relative) was found relevant for 37 cultures, but did not play a central role in these cultures, c) "contagion" (i.e. the contact with particular individuals, objects, and substances such as menstruation blood, menstruating women or deceased persons) was found for 49 cultures, d) "taboo violation" (most important of which are food taboos, sex taboos, verbal taboos like blasphemy, and sensory taboos, like taboos against touching or seeing something) that were found for 105 of all 139 cultures examined. Theories of *animistic causation* comprise "soul loss" and "spirit aggression" with the latter being most frequent and found in nearly all (137 of 139) cultures, 78 in which it is the predominant causal belief, especially in East Asia. Also common are theories of *magical causation*. Sorcery, i.e. the use of magic by humans, such as soul capture, necromancy, and use of hairs and nails to perform magic rites, and witchcraft, i.e. magic performed by witches and wizards, play a significant role in 72 cultures, too. Both, theories of animistic causation and sorcery (including the belief in the "evil eye", see below) can often be found around the Mediterranean, while witchcraft plays an important role in the Pacific area.

Studies focusing on illness beliefs in populations of Turkish origin

A few studies focus on illness perceptions in Turkish individuals, most of which are comparatively old.[4] They show that Turkish persons hold particular perceptions regarding their diseases, often facilitated by their Muslim belief.

Karanci (1986) surveyed 70 patients from a psychiatric clinic in urban Turkey regarding the causal attributions of their disease. She found out that to a large extent patients attributed natural causes to their disease. However, her 31-item instrument included only two items on supernatural causes which addressed bad luck and fate. This disproportion in item selection may have inadvertently biased the results. Similar findings were reproduced by the author some years later using the same instrument (Karanci 1993). Earlier studies by Öztürk (1964, 1965) came to different results showing the significant role of supernatural attributions, the most important of which were the will of God, obsession, and taboo violation. Nazar, i.e. the belief that a malicious glance of others can cause harm (also referred to as the "evil eye"), and sorcery have also been linked to disease and bad luck, infertility, and anxiety. Following this belief, accidents and diseases can be caused by jealousy and malevolence of others or by own violation of rules and rites (also see Yildirim-Fahlbusch 2003; Tilli 1989). Except for the IPQ-R validation study by Kocaman et al. (2007), no recent studies focus on illness beliefs in Turkey using a comprehensive framework. This could be changed in future by the availability of the Turkish IPQ-R. However, general studies of health and illness in Turkey suggest that supernatural causal attributions and control beliefs still play an important role (e.g., see Önder 2007).

In literature, two studies can be found that focus on Turkish migrant populations. Minas et al. (2007) surveyed 444 Turkish migrants residing in Melbourne with respect to their causal attributions. The authors applied the categories found by Murdock et al. (1978) by means of a self-made questionnaire. In their study, patients showed both

---

4   The results are based on a literature review whose methods are outlined in Appendix B.

natural and supernatural attributions to varying extents and different for different diseases. 62.8% of patients attributed physical stress and 69.0% attributed infections to somatic diseases. Critical life events and mental stress was most frequently mentioned for mental diseases (68.2% and 62.9%, respectively). However, for both illness groups also supernatural theories were important. One third of all patients held contagion, curses, or taboo violations responsible for physical disease. Additionally, more than 50% of patients held ominous sensations, taboo violation, and animistic causes such as soul loss responsible for mental diseases. Minas et al.'s analysis further showed that the attribution of natural instead of supernatural causes was associated with higher levels of education and acculturation to the country of origin. Also, persons with low self-perceived health status tended to attribute supernatural instead of natural causes to their diseases.

Franz et al. (2007) applied a modified version of the IPQ-R (different from Kocaman et al.'s version) in a sample of 79 Turkish patients of a psychiatric institution and compared their illness beliefs to matched German controls. Except for the Turkish validation study of the IPQ-R, it is the first and only quantitative assessment of illness beliefs using Leventhal's framework in a Turkish population. The study showed that Turkish patients had weaker control beliefs than German patients and held external factors more often responsible for their disease. Furthermore, Turkish patients were more thoroughly convinced of the chronicity and consequences of their disease.

4. Examining illness perceptions in migrants: A case study

In order to illustrate methodical challenges involved in the application of quantitative instruments in migrants, we used the research on illness perceptions as a case study. For this purpose we translated the Brief IPQ into Turkish and assessed the psychometric properties of the Turkish version of the IPQ-R (as provided by Kocaman et al. 2007) and the translated Brief IPQ in Turkish migrants residing in Germany. For the IPQ-R, divergent and structural validity as well as the internal consistency were determined. For the Brief IPQ, convergent and divergent validity were assessed.

Examining these validity types on an exploratory basis will also help to disclose starting points for an adaptation of the instruments to Turkish migrants and will allow to derive implications for a full-scale validation and further confirmatory research.

4.1 Methodical approach

4.1.1 Translation and adaptation of the Brief IPQ

The translation of the Brief IPQ followed published guidelines comprising a forward and backward translation (Beaton et al. 2000; van de Vijver/Hambleton 1996). However, for reasons of practicability and considering a limited time frame, the translation process was simplified (see Fig. 4).

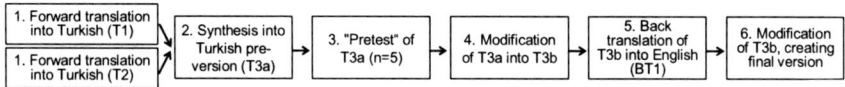

Fig. 4: Graphical representation of the Brief IPQ translation process (Source: Own illustration)

The principal investigator of the study was involved in each stage of the translation and documented results in writing. The Brief IPQ was independently translated by two translators with proficiency in Turkish, resulting in the two translations T1 and T2 (step 1). The translators then synthesized these translations into the pre-version T3a (step 2) that was pre-tested in five patients (three males, two females) (step 3). On the basis of these results, the instrument was slightly modified to improve understanding and to avoid ambiguity by simplifying and standardizing the wording (step 4). For example, the verb *hissetmek (to feel, to perceive)* was replaced by the verb *düşünmek* (to think) which is straight forward and consistent with its use in the other questions. Also, the word *semptomlar* was replaced by *belirtiler*. Although both mean "symptoms", the latter is more common in Turkish everyday language usage and was also used by the translators of the IPQ-R. Some respondents encountered problems with the 0-10 scaling proposed by the developers of the Brief IPQ. For them, it did not become clear that the scales represent an intensity rating between the two given and labeled endpoints. Because of this, we together with the translators decided to add additional instructions to the introductory part of the instrument explaining the response format. As another slight modification of the original version, we decided to present additional expressions of English words in brackets for which alternative phrases exist in Turkish language. These are the verb *kaygılanmak (to be concerned about)* complemented with the alternative *endişelenmek* having the same meaning, the adjective *net (clear)* complemented with the alternative *iyi (good)*, and the noun *ruh hali (mood, mental well being)* complemented with the alternative *duygu (feeling, sensation)*. Presenting both expressions helps to ensure that persons familiar with one phrase more than with the other understand the meaning of each item properly. This procedure is sometimes chosen in cultural adaptations of instruments to avoid misunderstanding (for example, cf. Gerritsen et al. 2004) and was also applied in the translation of the IPQ-R. The modified version (T3b) was back-translated by a third translator with proficiency in both Turkish and English (BT1) (step 5). Discrepancies between both versions were resolved. The adjective *korkak* in the last item was replaced by the adjective *kaygı*. Although both mean "anxious", "scared" or "afraid", the former is also used derogatively for "coward" in Turkish language (cf. English "chicken"). Furthermore, the example given in brackets for the last item was worded differently in order to use standard Turkish and an easier language style. Implementing these modifications, a final version was created (step 6).

4.1.2 Case study design

Inclusion and exclusion criteria

Turkish migrants with chronic diseases residing in Germany were included in the study. As described in chapter 2.3, the group of Turkish migrants is very heterogeneous and some are more proficient in German than in the Turkish language. Hence, Turkish language questionnaires cannot be administered to persons of Turkish descent without prior assessment of their language knowledge. For content-related research, experiences show that it is valid to choose the questionnaire language based on participants' preferences ("principle of free language choice") (e.g. Boos-Nünning 1986). Similarly, in the current study individuals were asked about their primary language and only those whose primary language was Turkish were included in the study. The level of proficiency in Turkish was not further assessed.

Patients came from different age and chronic illness groups. Individuals not capable of filling in questionnaires on their own due to little or no competency in writing and reading were not excluded from the study. Same as with individuals not able to fill in questionnaires on their own due to illness or disability, structured interviews were used as a method for questionnaire administration in this sub-group (see below). Methodical problems arising from the combination of different administration methods (self-administration and administration by means of structured interviews) were taken into account and will be discussed in chapter 4.3. Despite these concerns and the fact that both the IPQ-R and the Brief IPQ were developed to be used in self-administered questionnaire-based surveys, exclusion of these individuals was not

considered practical. Especially, the Brief IPQ is supposed to be used in clinical practice where it must be also valid for illiterate Turkish migrants. Hence, exclusion of illiterate persons from validation would impose considerable restrictions on its practical
value.

Recruitment and surveying of participants

Participants were recruited in self-help groups (SHGs) and rehabilitation clinics.

Self-help groups (SHGs)

In self-help groups, individuals were approached before, during, or after the sessions
and were asked to fill in questionnaires on the spot. Since these self-help groups tar-
geted women, no male participants could be surveyed in this setting. Illiterate women
or women not capable of filling in the questionnaire on their own for other reasons
were interviewed according to the procedure outlined above. The capability of filling
in self-administered questionnaires (SAQs) was assessed by means of self-report.
Hence, women could decide whether they preferred an interview or not. The inclusion criterion of chronic illness was assessed by means of self-report as well. All
women who participated in sessions during which recruitment took place were approached and asked if they liked to participate. Response rate was comparably low.
Of 35 women attending the sessions, only 19 (54.3%) participated. 10 of these had to
be interviewed by a member of the survey team due to illiteracy.

Rehabilitation clinics

Three rehabilitation clinics were selected for recruitment. Since 2000, they offer rehabilitation services tailored to Turkish language patients covering different diseases.
They aim at targeting particular needs for this patient group. This includes, among
other things, providing therapies through professionals that have the same sex as the
patient, offering therapies and exercises separately for men and women, offering
meals according to Muslim rules, and adjusting therapeutic regimens to Islamic
prayer times. In each clinic offering these services for Turkish migrants, one social
education worker proficient in Turkish language and of Turkish origin is employed
who coordinates therapies and acts as a mediator between Turkish patients and non-
Turkish personnel. These three persons (one in each of the three clinics) served as
contact persons and local coordinators and helped to organize the recruitment in the
setting.

Patients were surveyed during their stay in the clinic using an in-house approach
(see Freise 2003 for details). This approach has some methodical drawbacks, but
gains a better response rate than other approaches such as postal surveys. The local
coordinators were asked to identify all Turkish migrant patients currently participating
in in-patient rehabilitation disregarding the type of their disease. For each patient,
they took down the Turkish language proficiency level and invited all those whose
primary language was Turkish to participate in the interview. Some patients (n=4)
were not considered for recruitment due to physical impairment or cognitive limita-

tions. Their socio-demographic details were recorded. Aside from inviting patients to take part in the survey, the coordinating staff took care of premises and rescheduled the treatment plan to allow participants to spend time for participation. In the course of the 2.5-month recruitment period, only those patients were recruited and surveyed that stayed in the clinics on one of the six days on which recruitment took place. In total, 70 individuals were asked to participate, of which 63 agreed, resulting in a response rate of 90.0%. Of these, 46 patients had to be interviewed, while 17 answered questionnaires on their own.

A flowchart of participants recruited for the current study and included for analysis is given by Fig. 5.

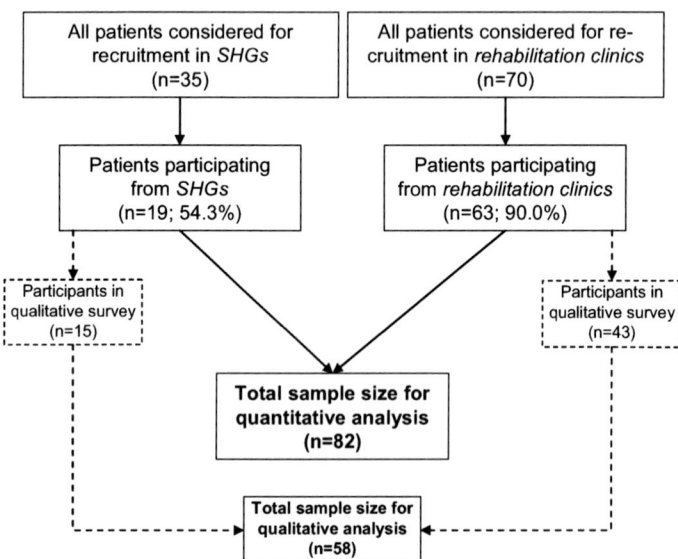

Fig. 5: Patient recruitment and study population included in the qualitative and quantitative analysis (Source: Own illustration)

4.1.3 Quantitative questionnaire and validation measures

The questionnaire instrument used

The questionnaire used for this study comprised the Turkish versions of the Medical Outcome Short Form Health Survey 12 (SF-12), followed by the revised version of the IPQ, the Positive and Negative Affect Schedule (PANAS), and the Brief IPQ. Additionally, few socio-demographic variables (e.g. sex, age, duration of illness measured by self-reported time in medical therapy, and duration of stay in Germany) were included. While the IPQ-R and the Brief IPQ were the primary instruments to be validated in this study, the SF-12 and PANAS were implemented as secondary instruments whose purpose was to make validation of the IPQ-R and the Brief IPQ possible. The questionnaire was accompanied by a cover letter briefly informing patients about the background of the study and emphasizing that participation in the study is voluntary and anonymous.

The Turkish version of the IPQ-R was slightly modified (see Appendix D for a version translated into English). This minor change comprised the inclusion of two additional causal attributions ("will of God" and "nazar") and the combination of the existing attributions "smoking" and "alcohol" into "smoking or alcohol". Furthermore, the word *koyunuz* in the instruction of the second part of the IPQ-R was replaced by *yapınız*, since the former is also used as a sexually connoted derogative and offensive term in colloquial Turkish. The last item of the Brief IPQ was deleted because it is (almost) identical to the last item of the IPQ-R. Kocaman et al. (2007) slightly changed the connotation of the response labels by using the verb *düşünmek (to think)* instead of *aynı fikirde olmak (to agree)*. This modification was retained.

The questionnaire was printed using both sides and a large font to ensure easy readability for older persons. Highlighting of rows further enhanced readability. Whereas in the version as provided by Kocaman et al. (2007) response categories for part II and III of the IPQ-R were numbered and listed in the instruction section of the respective parts, we decided to place categories directly above the check boxes. This is consistent with the layout of the original version of the IPQ-R and the other questions used in the research instrument.

Medical Outcome Short Form Health Survey 12 (SF-12)

The Medical Outcome Short Form Health Survey 12 (SF-12) was used as a measure of health-related quality of life (HRQOL). The SF-12 is a subset of the SF-36 (Ware et al. 1992) allowing the production of the same scores (physical and mental) as the full version (Ware et al. 1996). The SF-36 was developed in the 1970s as part of the Medical Outcome Study to assess health-related quality of life. Since then, it has become a well-tested instrument and has been frequently used in many national and international studies, in different population, and for different research questions including health economics. It has been standardized and translated for a number of different populations, coordinated by the International Quality of Life Assessment Group (IQOLA). Both the SF-36 and the SF-12 are generic instruments. Aside from assessing HRQOL, the SF-36 and its derivatives have been used in the examination of subjective health, considering social, mental, and physical aspects (Ware 2003).

The SF-36 consists of eight latent dimensions (Fig. 6). Together they form the two composite scale scores of physical (PCS) and mental health (MCS). Instead of 36 questions, the SF-12 uses only scores from a subset of 12 questions to compute these two scores, ranging from 0 to 100 with higher numbers representing better health. This allows for a more efficient and faster assessment of HRQOL, thus reducing test-taker burden. However, these advantages go at the cost of precision that is reduced by 10% and less accurate representation of the physical and mental dimension (Ware et al. 1996). Besides, with the SF-12 it is not possible to directly estimate the eight sub-domains provided by the SF-36, thus limiting comparability. In studies, the SF-12 proved to have a high test-retest reliability of 0.89 for PCS and 0.76 for MCS, adequate discriminatory power, and a good construct validity of 0.95 and 0.96 for PCS and MCS, respectively (ibid, see also the overview paper by the University of Wollongong 2005). For both instruments, versions for different purposes exist, differing in questionnaire type (self-report, external judgment, interview) as well as in the time period covered (4-week recall, acute 1-week, 24-hour recall). Apart from the 12-item version, an 8-item version (SF-8) exists. Unlike the former, this is not a subset of items of the SF-36, but a collection of newly developed single-item questions. Its psychometric properties are worse as compared to the other versions (Ware et al. 2001). No Turkish translation of the SF-8 is available (QualityMetric Inc. 2008).

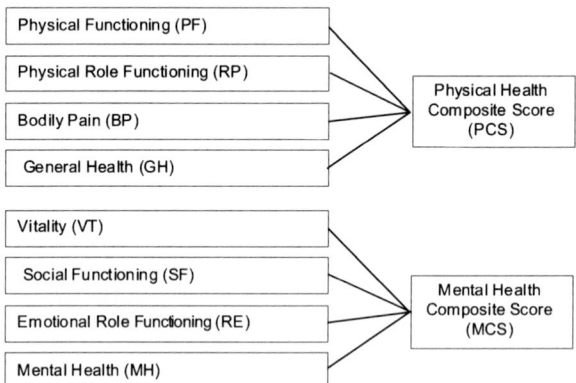

Fig. 6: Sub-domains and composite scores of the SF-36 (Source: Simplified visualization following Ware 2003)

For this case study, the Turkish version of the SF-12 was used. Unlike the full version that is validated and widely used in Turkish language *(Kısa Form 36)* (Koçyiğit et al. 1999; Pinar 2005), the Turkish version of the SF-12 has not been formally tested. However, since it merely is an item subset of the SF-36, it has been used in different studies (e.g. Akarçay et al. 2003; Reijneveld et al. 2003). Taking into account the amount of items already covered through the two IPQ questionnaires, we decided to apply the 12- instead of the 36-item version. Limitation of this approach will be discussed in chapter 4.3.5.

In 2000, a revision of the SF-36, the SF-36v2, has been published (Ware et al. 2000). Changes there also affect the SF-12 since it uses the SF-36 as a basis. Hence, also a new version of the SF-12, the SF-12v2, was created. Aside from changes in the layout, six-level responses of the last question that have been used in version 1 were changed into five-level responses to simplify items. Also, dichotomous responses in question 4 were changed into five-level responses. According to the authors (ibid), the SF-12v2 gains a better comparability with cultural and language adaptations used world-wide. Additionally, representing one of the major advantages, the SF-12v2 allows the estimation of the eight sub-domains shown in Fig. 6. Since the SF-36v2 has not been validated in Turkey, we applied version 1 of the SF-12. This approach is consistent with most other studies in Turkish populations that make use of this HRQOL instrument.

The first item of the SF-36 and the SF-12 on self-perceived health status (SPHS) is frequently used as a measure of general health (cf. Maddox/Douglas 1973), which was also the case in our study.

Positive and Negative Affect Schedule (PANAS)

The Positive and Negative Affect Schedule (PANAS) developed by Watson et al. (1988) was used to determine the divergent validity of the Turkish version of the IPQ-R and the Brief IPQ. The PANAS comprises a list of 20 different affects, 10 of which are positive (alert, active, attentive, determined, enthusiastic, excited, inspired, interested, proud, strong) and 10 of which are negative (afraid, ashamed, distressed, guilty, hostile, irritable, jittery, nervous, scared, upset). They form the two dimensions "Positive Affects" (PA) and "Negative Affects" (NA). Respondents are asked to rate the intensity of these feelings (ranging from 1 = "very slightly or not at all" to 5 = "extremely") during the past week. In this way, it measures the degree of activity and alertness on the one hand and distress and discomfort on the other hand. Research shows that the instrument has sufficient reliability, stability over time, and that the two scales are uncorrelated (ibid). The instrument has been translated into Turkish *(Pozitif ve Negatif Duygu Ölçeği)* and validated by Gençöz (2000), showing properties consistent with the original version. It was used as provided by that author.

Questionnaire administration

Self-administered (SAQ) vs. interviewer-administered questionnaires (IAQ)

Studies in health research relaying on self-reports through self-administered instruments may be faced with different problems. As mentioned above, studies on ethnic minorities face the problem that many of these individuals have little or no reading and writing competencies. This is also true for Turkish migrants residing in Germany. Especially, the first generation of these migrants has received little formal education in their home country. This is particularly the case for first-generation Turkish women, whose illiteracy rates are higher than in their male counterparts (Ucar 1996). Hence, the application of self-report measures should not be restricted to self-administered questionnaires but, for some individuals, must alternatively offer structured interviews. Within structured interviews (also known as standardized interviews, interviewer-administered or researcher-administered questionnaires or surveys) each participant is asked the same set of questions orally, using the same wording and question order (Arthur/Nazroo 2003). This technique was also applied in the current study as an alternative to self-administration thus resulting in a dual mixed-mode assessment. Responses to each question were written down by the interviewer. Hence, the procedure is very similar to self-administered questioning with the difference that questions are read aloud and answers are communicated orally. Structured interviews can be regarded as the best alternative when self-administration is not possible and are also applied in other validations studies, as shows an unsystematic search in the major data bases. Hence, it was also used for the current study as an alternative method when subjects were not able (or not willing) to fill in questionnaires on their own.

Examining the usability of the questionnaire

Aside from the quantitative survey, a qualitative survey on the usability of the questionnaire compilation was carried out by means of structured interviews. For this survey, all participants recruited in self-help groups and rehabilitation clinics were interviewed by the interviewers with respect to their opinion about the questionnaire. Interviews followed quantitative assessment and were recorded in writing by the research team. Standardized open-ended questions asked participants to describe the difficulty and their impression of the questionnaire (including its layout), to identify ambiguous words and wordings, to judge the appropriateness of the Turkish language and style used, as well as to make suggestions for improvement. Interviews were conducted in Turkish. A structured topic guide was used (see Appendix E) to standardize both content as well as the order of questions in which persons were interviewed, thus to reduce the influence of context effects. These can arise when the response behavior of individuals is influenced by the way and/or order in which questions are asked. Since context effects very seldom can be eliminated, it is important to hold their impact constant across the entire study population. Using standardized topic guides contributes to this purpose (Brace/Adams 2006).

The majority of patients recruited in the clinics and SHGs took also part in the qualitative survey. In the clinics, 20 patients could not take the qualitative survey due to other obligations such as appointments. In the self-help groups, 4 patients did not want to participate (Fig. 5). Answers were translated by the research team and categorized according to their contents. Analyses followed the approach of qualitative content analysis by Mayring (2000).

4.1.4 Composite measures and imputation of missing values

Different composite measures were calculated for the IPQ-R, the SF-12 and PANAS according to published guidelines of the respective instruments. Scoring of the SF-12 MCS and PCS was done by means of a SAS algorithm modified to comply with SPSS syntax language. It was based on instructions published by Ware et al. (1995) and applied standard weighting that was considered sufficient for this study. To calculate the positive (PA) and negative affect (NA) dimensions, respective items were summed-up. For PA these were the items F1, F3, F5, F9, F10, F12, F14, F16, F17, F19; for NA the remaining items F2, F4, F6, F7, F8, F11, F13, F15, F18, F20 of the PANAS; with higher rates (minimum 10, maximum 50 for each of the two dimensions) indicating stronger positive and negative affect, respectively. For part II of the IPQ-R, standard item assignment and dimensions as proposed by Moss-Morris et al. (2002) were used. Item assignment for part III was slightly adjusted to comply with the changes made. Hence, the attributions "nazar" and "God's will" were intended to add to the existing "chance/accident" dimension, while "smoking or alcohol" were intended to be part of the "risk factor" attribution. However, this issue was also subject to further analysis and will be taken up in chapter 4.2. Dimensions and respective item numbers for part II and III of the IPQ-R are shown in Tab. 3.

Dimension	Range	Items
Part II: Core beliefs about illness		
Timeline acute/chronic (TLA)	6-30	C1*, C2[5], C3, C4*, C5, C18*
Timeline cyclical (TLC)	4-20	C29, C30, C31, C32
Consequences (CSQ)	6-30	C6, C7, C8*, C9, C10, C11
Personal Control (PCR)	6-30	C12, C13, C14, C15*, C16, C17*
Treatment Control (TCR)	5-25	C19*, C20, C21, C22, C23*
Illness Coherence (ILC)	5-25	C24*, C25*, C26*, C27*, C28
Emotional representations (ERP)	6-30	C33, C34, C35, C36*, C37, C38
Part III: Causal attributions		
Psychological attributions (PSY-CA)	6-30	D1, D9, D10, D11, D12, D17
Risk factor attributions (RF-CA)	5-25	D2, D4, D6, D8, D13, D15
Immune attributions (IMM-CA)	3-15	D3, D7, D18
Chance/accident attributions (CHA-CA)	4-20	D5, D14, D16, D19

Note. * item reversed

Tab. 3: Coding of the IPQ part II and III dimensions (Source: Own illustration)

As shown in the table above, reversed scoring was used for some items in harmony with the original English version. Scale measures were calculated by summing up item scores in each dimension as proposed by Moss-Morris et al. (2002). Since each dimension consists of a different number of items, the range of possible scores is varying between the seven dimensions with higher scores indicating stronger representations.

Imputation algorithms for missing values

Some statistical methods applied in this study, e.g. factor analysis, involve a large number of variables and cannot deal with missing values. Instead, cases with one or more missing values in one of the variables involved in the computation process usually are automatically excluded from analysis. Except for a selection bias not to be neglected, this problem could be tolerated in studies in which the sample size is large enough to compensate for these "lost" cases. In studies with small sample sizes, the problem of selection bias is accompanied by an underpowering of the analysis that in some cases can even make available data incompatible with requirements and assumptions of statistical procedures. For instance, as outlined in the method section, 80 cases were set as the minimum requirement to perform factor analysis of the 38 variables of the IPQ-R part II. However, since 34 out of 82 cases had missing values in one or more of the 38 variables (see chapter 4.2), this would

---

5   See Appendix D. "C" refers to the section of the quantitative questionnaire applied in this study. "2" designates the item number. This notation will also be used in other chapters of this paper.

reduce the number of cases available to perform factor analysis to 48 and clearly violate basic requirements for this statistical procedure. Hence, it was necessary to impute missing values. Imputation as such is a step often performed in studies for statistical procedures where a large number of variables is involved and that do not allow to operate with undefined values, i.e. missings, in data cells. Aside from factor analysis, this is for instance the case in regression analysis or in the calculation of composite measures (Munro 2005). Because of this necessity, for many popular instruments, imputation instructions exist. These are usually accompanied by sensitivity studies showing that analyses performed on imputed data fulfilling certain requirements produce results similar to analyses on complete data. Respective imputation strategies and sensitivity studies also exist for most of the instruments applied in this study. The imputation procedure used for each of the four instruments will be described in the following.

SF-12

Since the algorithm developed by Ware et al. (1995) to calculate the two composite measures PCS and MCS utilizes all variables, scale measures can not be computed for cases with missing values in one or more of these 12 items. As Perneger/Burnand (2005) have shown, it is possible to impute up to three missing values per dimension (PCS and MCS) of the SF-12 by means of a simple algorithm without causing serious problems with loss of data quality. This algorithm substitutes each missing value by the mean sample weights applied to the calculation of the PCS and MCS.

PANAS

As described previously, the two composite measures of the PANAS are calculated by summing up respective items. The authors of the instrument proposed a simple formula to deal with the situation of missing values: In case one or more missings exist among the summands, the sum for PA and NA, respectively, is calculated as 10 (i.e. the number of items per each of the two scales) divided by the number of non-missing items of this scale multiplied by the sum of these non-missing items (Watson et al. 1988).

IPQ-R

For imputation, Frostholm et al. (2005) proposed a procedure based on regression. Instead of imputing the items the respective scales consists of, Frostholm et al.'s procedure estimates scale scores based on the best subset regression. Aside from the other illness perceptions sum scores, the authors included illness worry, emotional distress, and socio-demographic variables as covariates into their model. A similar approach was used in this study. However, instead of emotional distress and illness worry, health-related quality of life was included into the model. Additionally, missings were only imputed for IPQ-R scales of which at least 2 items were non-missing. The same procedure was applied to the scales examining causal attributions (IPQ part III).

Brief IPQ

Imputation becomes more difficult the fewer items a scale consists of (Huisman 2000). Among the five studies that applied the Brief IPQ up to now, none made use of an imputation strategy for missing values. Since the number of missings among the nine Brief IPQ items was comparably low in the current study (see chapter 4.2), missings were not imputed either.

4.1.5 Validation process and statistical analysis

The validation process of the *IPQ-R* included several steps.

Validity of the IPQ-R part I

Validity of the identity subscale was tested in two ways: First, by comparing the mean of the subscales assessing identity and experienced symptoms, and second by calculating the proportion of symptoms that are part of patients' identity with disease.

Structural validity of the IPQ-R part II and III

Although confirmatory factor analysis (CFA) is considered the gold-standard for factor structures that are known from previous research (Hu/Bentler 1999), an exploratory approach was used in this study in order to assess structural validity of part II and III of the IPQ-R. In general, exploratory factor analysis (EFA) is regarded as requiring a smaller sample size than CFA and is therefore suitable for a pilot study (Kline 2005; Marsh et al. 1998). There is a controversy about how large this sample size should be and whether the sample size per se or the ratio of the total number of cases to the number of items is crucial. Guidelines vary heavily from n=50 to n>1000 for the former and <5:1 to >30:1 for the latter (Osborne/Costello 2004). These rules of thumb lack any empirical basis (MacCallum et al. 1999). In a newer publication, Sapnas/Zeller (2002) on the basis of their calculations state that a total number of 50 to 100 cases is sufficient to perform exploratory factor analysis. To be parsimonious and to meet the philosophy of a pilot study (a "miniature version" of the actual project) but none the less be able to perform EFA for testing purposes, in this study, a sample size of at least n=80 was chosen.

In line with previous research on methodical aspects of the IPQ-R (e.g. Moss-Morris et al. 2002), principal component analysis (PCA) with Kaiser normalized varimax rotation was chosen (Bühner 2006) as the extraction method. Different measures were applied to examine whether requirements to perform factor analysis were met:

The *Kaiser-Meyer-Olkin (KMO)* coefficient allows a first judgment whether the variable selection is suitable to be considered for factor analysis. This coefficient represents the common variance shared by all variables divided by the common variance shared by all variables plus their partial correlation coefficients. KMO coefficients below 0.5 indicate a variable set incompatible with factor analysis (Tabachnick/Fidell 1996; Bühner 2006).

The *anti-image correlation matrix* contains the negative partial correlations of the items and designates the proportion of the variance that is independent from other variables. Ideally, most or all of the values below the MSA diagonal (see chapter 4.2.2 for an actual application) should be as small as possible, preferably close to zero (ibid).

Similarly, the *measure of sample adequacy (MSA)* can be applied. It tells about the partial correlation between one item and the remaining items. It should be interpreted in a similar way as the KMO coefficient. Unlike the latter, the MSA does not take the adequacy of the entire correlation matrix into account but allows a statement about the compatibility of each item with the given factor structure. As a rule of thumb, variables with values below 0.5 can be considered not fitting the factor structure properly (ibid; Kaiser and Rice 1974).

Finally, *Bartlett's test of sphericity* tests the null hypothesis that all correlations are close to zero. Hence a significant test indicates that variables are sufficiently correlated to perform factor analysis (Tabachnick/Fidell 1996; Bühner 2006).

Apart from these, *other criteria* exist to extract an optimal number of factors (ibid). Since this study aimed to confirm or reject the structures identified by the other IPQ-R validation studies, the number of factors to extract was pre-set to 7 for part II and to 4 for part III of the IPQ-R (cf. Moss-Morris et al. 2002, Kocaman et al. 2007, and Giardini et al. 2007). For reasons outlined in chapter 4.2.2, in addition, scree plots (Catell 1966), the original and the revised minimum average partial test (MAP) as well as parallel analysis (O'Connor 2000) were applied to find an alternative factor structure for part III of the IPQ-R.

As an additional measure of structural validity, the *item discrimination power* within each dimension has been calculated and illustrated as corrected item-total correlation coefficients (r_{itc}). These coefficients give the correlation of each item and the respective scale they belong to, with this item considered not a part of this scale. This corrects for a spurious inflation of the respective items that would emerge if items would be calculated twice in the computation of the correlation coefficients. Items with item-total correlation coefficients below 0.3 can be considered problematic in terms of factorability (Bühner 2006).

To stay conservative, Spearman r_s was used as a measure of correlation to assess the relationship between dimensions. Furthermore, the relationship of the IPQ-R and the SF-12 MCS and PCS dimensions was analyzed by the same means. To assess the relationship of IPQ-R items among each other, Pearson correlation coefficients have been calculated, since they also form the basis for factor analytical algorithms. Items were regarded as quasi-metric.

Divergent validity and internal reliability of the IPQ part II and III

Divergent validity was tested by analyzing the correlation between IPQ-R subscales and the positive and negative affect dimension of the PANAS and the two dimensions of the SF-12 (IPQ-R part II only). Internal consistency was measured using Cronbach's α.

Validity of the Brief IPQ

The Brief IPQ was validated by comparing answers to answers in the IPQ-R using correlation coefficients (convergent validity) and by applying the PANAS and SF-12 (divergent validity) as mentioned above.

Other statistical aspects

To stay conservative, the non-parametric Mann-Whitney-U- and Kruskal-Wallis-H-test were carried out to analyze differences in quasi-metric variables between groups. The Shapiro-Wilk-W-test was applied to test for the normality of distributions. All statistical tests were two-sided with a significance level set to 0.05 if not mentioned otherwise. Tests for multiple comparisons were Bonferroni corrected (Hinton 2004). Data was analyzed using SPSS for Windows version 15 (SPSS Inc. 2006).

4.2   Validity and usability of the instruments

In the following, the results of the case study will be presented. Following a description of the sample and a missing value analysis, descriptive statistics and distributions of items and scales will be outlined, and the results of the pilot validation process presented. Finally, on the basis of the qualitative survey, this chapter will elaborate on the usability of the IPQ-R and the Brief IPQ in the sample of Turkish migrants.

4.2.1 Description of the sample

Socio-demographics and illness groups

In total, the sample consisted of 82 cases, 19 (23.2%) of which were surveyed in SHGs and 63 (76.8%) of which were surveyed in clinics. Tab. 4 shows some basic characteristics of the study sample stratified by sex and study site.

	Sex		Study site		Total
	Male (n=34)	Female (n=48)	Self-help groups (n=19)	Rehabilitation clinics (n=63)	(n=82)
Sex					
Male (%)			0.0	54.0	41.5
Female (%)			100.0	46.0	58.5
Administration type					
Self-administered (%)	50.0	56.3	47.4	49.2	53.7
Self-administered /w assistance (%)	8.8	8.3	5.3	9.5	8.5
Interviewer-administered (%)	41.2	35.4	47.4	41.3	37.8
Age (x̄ ; s)	55.6;11.2	50.2;12.2	50.9; 12.9	52.9;11.7	52.4; 11.9

Tab. 4: Basic characteristics stratified by sample, sex, and study site (Source: Own data)

Due to the different indications the study sites were specialized in, the sample comprised patients suffering from various illnesses. As shown in Tab. 5, five different illness groups could be identified with most patients suffering from cardiovascular diseases[6]. Patients suffering from illness other than these five major conditions were collapsed into a sixth category labeled "other physical diseases" comprising, among other things, renal disease and arthrosis.

Disease:	Diabetes (n=12)	Cardio-vascular (n=33)	Respira-tory (n=6)	Cancer (n=7)	Mental (n=8)	Other physical (n=16)
Sex						
Male (%)	58.3	48.5	50.0	28.6	12.5	31.3
Female (%)	41.7	51.5	50.0	71.4	87.5	68.7
Administration type						
Self-administered (%)	58.3	48.5	50.0	14.3	62.5	75.0
Self-administered /w assistance (%)	0.0	3.0	16.7	14.3	37.5	6.3
Interviewer-administered (%)	41.7	48.5	33.3	71.4	0.0	18.7
Age ($\bar{x}$; s)	55.7;11.3	57.4;8.8	55.7;15.0	56.0;8.4	42.3;12.5	42.0;9.5
Duration of illness ($\bar{x}$; s)	9.8;10.6	8.1;8.9	14.1;10.7	1.1;1.0	6.0;8.6	7.5;8.0
Self-rated health ($\bar{x}$; s)	4.0;0.7	3.9;0.7	3.7;0.5	3.7;0.5	4.3;0.5	3.3;0.8

Tab. 5: Characteristics of the different illness groups (Source: Own data)

Corresponding with the male-female ratio in the total sample and the composition of the self-help groups, the proportion of females also exceeded the proportion of males in three illness groups. No significant differences in sex ratio existed in the largest (cardiovascular diseases, n=33) and the smallest illness group (respiratory diseases, n=6). Men only predominated in the diabetes group. Other socio-demographic and general characteristics differed between the six strata as well: on average, patients with mental diseases and patients categorized in the collapsed group "other physical diseases" were considerably younger (mean difference approximately 13-15 years) than patients from other illness groups. These younger groups also consisted of proportionally less persons not able or willing to fill in questionnaires on their own. In these groups, all or more than four-fifth, respectively, of individuals filled in questionnaires alone or with little assistance by the research team. Rates of self-administration or assisted self-administration ranged from 28.6 to 66.7% in the other groups. Illness durations varied significantly across groups (p<0.05). The self-perceived health status applied as a measure of general health showed little variation between the six groups, ranging from 3.33 and 4.33 on the quasi-metric five-point scale (1="excellent health"; 5="bad health"). The only significant difference in self-rated health existed between patients with mental conditions and patients collapsed into "other physical diseases" that showed the best health status among all illness groups (Bonferroni-corrected p<0.05).

---

6   Some of the resulting groups, particularly respiratory diseases (n=6), cancer (n=7), and mental diseases (n=8), are very small in sample size. Therefore, all calculations stratifying by illness groups as presented in the following, must be treated with caution.

Missing value analysis

Sex, age, type of illness, study site, one item of the Brief IPQ, and two items of the second part of the IPQ-R were the only variables that had been filled in by all patients of the sample. Other items showed a varying number of missing values. Most can be found in the items asking patients whether symptoms they experienced since the beginning of their illness (right-hand side of part I of the IPQ-R examining illness identity; see Appendix C.1) are associated with their disease. These 14 items were skipped by about 26.8 to up to 46.3% of persons surveyed hinting at some severe problems, being also in line with observations made during the qualitative survey and described in interviewer reports (see chapter 4.2.3). The range of missing values for the left-hand site of the IPQ-R part was 6.1 to 19.5%.

The proportion of missing values in *part II* of the IPQ-R ranged from 0 to 11.0% (Fig. 7). Taking into account the underlying latent structures of these items, it becomes evident that the proportion of missing values was unequal over the seven IPQ-R dimensions. While for emotional representations (C33-C38), consequences (C6-C11), and timeline cyclical (C29-C32) no item exceeded a missing value proportion of 5%, this proportion was higher for the remaining dimensions and highest for personal control (C12-C17) where all but one item had more than 7.5% missing values among all responses for these items.

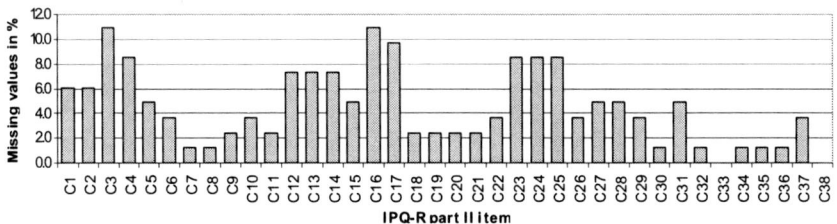

Fig. 7: Proportion of missing values in part II of the IPQ-R (Source: Own data)

Missing values for *part III* items on causal attribution ranged from 1.2% to 11.0% as shown in Fig. 8, with diet (item 4) and own behavior (item 8) having the most missings among all responses (11.0%). Fewer people omitted answers in the *Brief IPQ* as can be seen in Fig. 9 where all nine items had less than 5% missing values.

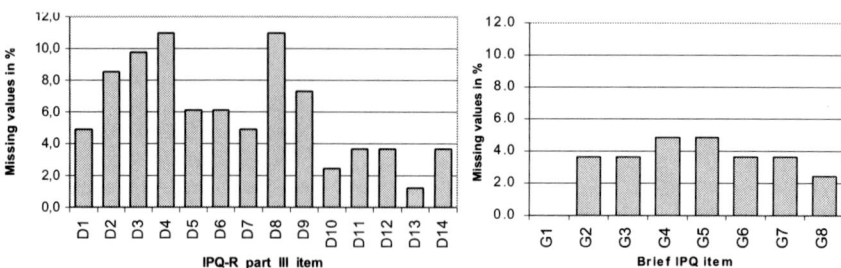

Fig. 8: Proportion of missing values in part III of the IPQ-R (Source: Own data)

Fig. 9: Proportion of missing values in the Brief IPQ (Source: Own data)

In the *SF-12*, proportion of missing values ranged from 2.4% for item 8 and 11.0% for item 3. 5 patients omitted more than 3 responses among the 6 key items for each the PCS and the MCS of the SF-12. In the *PANAS* instrument, number of missing values was comparably low and <5% for all items. No clear missing value pattern became evident in the four instruments when the matrix of missings by cases and variables was examined (not shown).

Imputation of missing values

As outlined in chapter 4.1.4, imputation algorithms were applied to each of the four instruments to reduce the number of missing values. Only 60 cases provided valid responses for all items of the SF-12. Since the computation of the two composite measures PCS and MCS utilizes all variables, this would have reduced the number of valid cases to 73.2% of the total sample size. By applying the algorithm above, all but five incomplete data rows could be imputed. The remaining 5 cases had more than 3 missing values among the SF-12 variables and were therefore not eligible for imputation following the strategy outlined above. Hence, for these cases, no composite measures were calculated and PCS and MCS were set to "missing" instead. 20 cases had incomplete data on the 20 items of the PANAS that are needed to calculate the positive and the negative affect score, limiting the available sample size to 75.6% of the total sample size. By applying imputation strategies, summery measures for all 20 cases with missing variables could be calculated resulting in complete information on PA and NA. 34 participants had missing values in one of the 38 items of part II and 23 items of part III of the IPQ-R. By using the imputation method described above, all seven summary measures of part II could be calculated for all but 2 cases. Data on the four dimensions of part III was available for 77 of 82 cases. Since many missing values existed in part I of the IPQ-R hinting at substantial problems of the scale, no imputation was performed here.

Univariate statistics and item distribution of the SF-12 and PANAS

SF-12

Physical and mental composite scores as measured by the SF-12 are shown in Tab. 6.

	Diabetes		Cardio-vasc.		Respiratory		Cancer		Mental		Other		Total	
	x̄	s	x̄	s	x̄	s	x̄	s	x̄	s	x̄	s	x̄	s
PCS	33.4	5.6	33.5	6.1	36.1	7.6	37.3	9.3	30.7	5.3	42.9	9.9	35.7	8.1
MCS	39.0	11.1	42.4	10.2	40.9	6.4	44.7	7.4	31.8	9.6	43.2	5.6	41.4	9.3

Tab. 6: SF-12 physical (PCS) and mental (MCS) composite measure stratified by illness groups (Source: Own data)

No significant differences between the groups regarding mental HRQOL existed as revealed an H-test corrected for multiple comparisons. "Other diseases" were significantly different from cardio-vascular diseases and mental conditions regarding PCS (Bonferroni-corrected p<0.05).

PANAS

The positive affect measure did not show significant differences between illness groups. Values ranged from 14 to 43 over all individuals with an average score of x̄=27.2. The range was wider for the negative affect score (10 to 46; x̄=20.7), significantly (p<0.05) varying between illness groups (Tab. 7).

	Diabetes		Cardio-vasc.		Respiratory		Cancer		Mental		Other		Total	
	x̄	s	x̄	s	x̄	s	x̄	s	x̄	s	x̄	s	x̄	s
PA	27.9	5.1	27.0	5.9	24.4	5.7	25.6	5.6	27.8	7.3	28.8	7.4	27.2	6.2
NA	24.3	8.1	19.8	8.6	15.2	4.7	14.7	2.9	26.8	7.6	21.4	6.7	20.7	8.0

Tab. 7: PANAS positive (PA) and negative (NA) affect stratified by illness groups (Source: Own data)

4.2.2 Validity of the IPQ-R

IPQ-R part I

The validity and reliability of the identity scale should have been tested by comparing the left- and right-hand subscale. However, since almost 50% of the respondents did not answer the right-hand side of the identity scale, a sound comparison was not possible. Analysis of the remaining cases with valid responses on both subscales revealed that correspondence between both was high (data not shown).

IPQ-R part II

Structural validity and scale distribution

A correlation matrix of items belonging to part II of the IPQ is shown in Tab. A 3. Since items, in line with expectations, correlated to varying degrees with each other with no items showing strong correlations above 0.8, basic requirements for factor analysis are met. In order to validate the factor structure of the second part of the IPQ-R and to confirm the factor structure found in the validation studies of the original and the translated version of the IPQ-R, principal component analysis (PCA) of all 38 items was performed. The Kaiser-Meyer-Olkin coefficient of the item set was 0.57, indicating that a considerable proportion of item variance is not shared by other items, thus revealing that the choice of items is not optimal, however border-line acceptable. This can be further analyzed by examining the anti-image correlation matrix and the measure of sample adequacy (MSA) (Tab. A 4). Ideally, most or all of the values off the diagonal (shaded in gray) should preferably be close to zero. As can be seen, this is not the case across all variables, indicating some misfit. Similarly, the MSA can be used to judge sample adequacy. Variables with values below 0.5 can be considered not fitting the factor structure properly. This is the case for several items as shown in the table (in bold face). Under a scale developing approach—that was not the purpose of this study—, removing these items would increase KMO significantly and improve the factor solution. Despite the small sample size, Bartlett's test of sphericity was significant ($p<0.001$), indicating that items are sufficiently correlated to perform factor analysis.

Setting the factor extraction criterion to an eigenvalue >1 as recommended in literature (cf. chapter 4.1.5) revealed a 10-factor solution (result not shown). By limiting the number of factors to 7 according to the original solution and replicated by other authors as outlined previously, the following factor loadings for the 7 dimensions were reached (Tab. 8).

IPQ-R part II dimensions/items	Factors							r_{itc}	α if deleted
	1	2	3	4	5	6	7		
Timeline acute/chronic (TLA), n=76, α=0.57									
C1: My illness will last a short time	-.01	.40	-.31	-.15	-.03	.30	.17	.10	.61
C2: My illness is likely to be permanent rather than temporary	-.04	-.07	.02	.04	.82	-.11	.07	.32	.51
C3: My illness will last a long time	.00	.03	-.10	.15	.85	-.03	.03	.49	.44
C4: This illness will pass quickly	.14	.36	-.47	.12	.35	.12	.16	.43	.46
C5: I expect to have this illness for the rest of my life	.11	.14	.27	-.17	.56	.06	.37	.35	.50
C18: My illness will improve in time	.06	.13	-.17	-.57	.19	.37	-.26	.18	.57
Timeline cyclical (TLC,), n=82, α=0.36									
C29: The symptoms of my illness change from day to day	.57	.14	.25	.17	-.04	-.08	.12	.32	.14
C30: My symptoms come and go in circles	.09	-.26	.42	.01	.27	-.11	-.01	.06	.44
C31: My illness is very unpredictable	.36	-.36	.06	-.09	-.06	-.12	-.23	.21	.27
C32: I go through cycles in which my illness gets better and worse	.62	.20	.18	-.12	.24	.23	-.02	.19	.29
Consequences (CSQ), n=82, α=0.71									
C6: My illness is a serious condition	.08	.11	.38	-.31	.40	.05	.35	.49	.67
C7: My illness has major consequences on my life	.43	.44	.30	-.23	.38	-.02	.16	.49	.67
C8: My illness does not have much effect on my life	.16	.59	.14	-.18	.24	-.17	-.10	.18	.75
C9: My illness strongly affects the way other see me	.39	-.24	-.15	-.02	.23	.10	.48	.34	.71
C10: My illness has serious financial consequences	.26	-.06	.04	-.01	.10	.03	.75	.53	.65
C11: My illness causes difficulties for those who are close to me	.36	.00	.16	.00	.14	-.25	.75	.68	.60
Personal Control (PCR), n=80, α=0.59									
C12: There is a lot I can do to control my illness	-.01	-.07	.68	.17	-.04	.18	.17	.46	.49
C13: What I do can determine whether my illness gets better or worse	.06	.33	.66	.18	.13	.04	.05	.56	.45
C14: The course of my illness depends on me	-.14	-.02	.81	.15	-.01	-.10	-.09	.48	.47
C15: Nothing I do will affect my illness	-.10	.80	.05	.18	-.02	.17	-.07	.21	.60
C16: I have the power to influence my illness	.16	-.42	.49	.24	.04	.22	.20	.22	.59
C17: My actions will have no effect on the outcome of my illness	-.03	.56	-.07	-.10	.03	.19	-.01	.10	.64
Treatment Control (TCR), n=80, α=0.70									
C19: There is very little that can be done to improve my illness	-.08	.51	-.15	.33	-.33	.01	-.10	.33	.70
C20: Treatment will be effective in treating my illness	.14	-.10	.31	.67	.05	.08	.17	.34	.69
C21: The neg. effects of my illness can be prevented by my treatment	-.13	.02	.08	.82	.04	.03	-.08	.63	.57
C22: Treatment can control my illness	.15	.17	.23	.69	.24	.16	-.23	.53	.62
C23: There is nothing that can help my illness	-.24	.49	-.09	.47	-.14	.05	-.16	.47	.65
Illness Coherence (ILC), n=80, α=0.72									
C24: The symptoms of my illness are puzzling to me	-.56	.11	.10	.01	.02	.39	-.06	.45	.69
C25: My illness has no meaning to me	-.06	.13	-.04	-.17	-.15	.72	.07	.52	.67
C26: I don't understand my illness	-.20	.11	.04	.15	-.07	.78	-.06	.68	.60
C27: My illness doesn't make any sense to me	-.34	.37	-.10	.13	-.04	.59	.03	.58	.64
C28: I have a clear picture or understanding of my illness	.14	-.17	.26	.17	.28	.55	-.19	.23	.77
Emotional representations (ERP), n=82, α=0.69									
C33: I get depressed when I think about my illness	.80	-.05	.02	.01	.06	-.12	.05	.72	.55
C34: When I think about my illness I get upset	.83	-.01	-.12	-.02	.05	-.15	.08	.81	.52
C35: My illness makes me feel angry	.64	.00	-.17	.01	-.06	-.26	.28	.59	.59
C36: My illness does not worry me	-.41	.08	-.23	-.06	.12	.01	-.19	-.36	.86
C37: My illness makes me feel anxious	.75	-.12	-.05	.01	.04	.05	.06	.58	.61
C38: My illness makes me feel afraid	.69	-.10	-.05	-.14	.08	.06	.23	.50	.63

Tab. 8: Principal component analysis (rotated solution) and internal consistency of IPQ-R part II items (Source: Own data)

While items of the dimensions on emotional representations, illness coherence, and treatment control performed acceptably as regards their factor loadings, the scales on consequences, timeline acute/chronic, and timeline cyclical consisted of many weak loadings, indicating that these factors, pre-set basing on the original publication, were not optimally represented by the given items in the current study. Also, high cross-loading existed (underscored), of which some exceeded the primary loadings. Item-total correlation coefficients (r_{itc}) were calculated as an additional measure of structural validity. As shown in Tab. 8, some items remained under the threshold of 0.3 meaning that these items share less than 9% (0.3*0.3) of variance with their respective summary scores and can be considered as problematic regarding their contribution to the internal consistency of the scale. The items "C30: My symptoms come and go in circles", "C1: My illness will last a short time", and "C17: My actions will have no effect on the outcome of my illness" performed worse regarding their discrimination power and just shared 0.36%, 1.0%, and 1.0% of variance, respectively, with the factors they belong to. The item "C36: My illness does not worry me" sufficiently represented the emotional representations scale (r_{itc}=-0.36). However, same as the respective factor loading of -0.41, the coefficient was negative, giving rise to the suspicion that the reversed poling of the item has been misunderstood by respondents. The low discrimination power of these items affects measurement accuracy which is also reflected in the internal consistency of the scale. It varied across dimensions and was $\alpha \geq 0.7$ for illness coherence, treatment control and consequences, and 0.69 for emotional representations. It was borderline acceptable for personal control (α=0.59) and timeline/acute chronic (α=0.57) and was very weak for timeline cyclical (α=0.36), corresponding with the low factor loadings of the four respective items. The negative impact of items with low discrimination power on scale homogeneity was also reflected in the α-if-item-deleted values for each item. They showed that the internal consistency of the IPQ-R dimension could be improved for the current population if certain items were deleted.

Under a scale development framework and a research question aiming at developing an instrument to assess illness beliefs, the corrected item-total correlation, α-if-item-deleted values, the measurement of sample adequacy, the indices of the anti-image correlation matrix, as well as additional measures of item analysis based on raw item scores, such as the analysis of item difficulty and item dispersion, as well as their ratios with item discrimination could be also used for the purpose of construction or for the refinement of a given instrument. This was not the purpose of the current study. However, these scale building measurements of which some have been presented just now help derive additional information about the performance of items in the current population.

Taking the factor structure shown above as a basis and defining the same dimensions as was done in other validation studies of the IPQ-R, it becomes evident that the distributions of 4 out of 7 factors (timeline acute/chronic, timeline cyclical, consequences, and personal control) resemble normal distributions (Fig. A 1 in Appendix A). These graphical impressions are further supported by the non-significant Shapiro-Wilks-tests for these dimensions, testing the null hypotheses that distributions do not differ from a normal distribution.

Scores of the respective dimensions were quite similar between the 5 groups of physical illness and slightly differed in comparison to mental diseases (Tab. 9). However, there were no statistically significant differences when significance tests were Bonferroni-corrected for multiple testing.

	Diabetes		Cardio-vasc.		Respiratory		Cancer		Mental		Other		Total	
	$\bar{x}$	s	$\bar{x}$	s	$\bar{x}$	s	$\bar{x}$	s	$\bar{x}$	s	$\bar{x}$	s	$\bar{x}$	s
TLA	18.6	4.7	20.3	5.0	19.0	6.5	18.8	2.7	20.4	4.0	19.9	4.0	19.8	4.6
TLC	13.1	3.4	13.6	3.5	13.5	2.4	15.3	2.4	14.5	2.3	12.0	2.3	13.4	3.1
CSQ	17.7	4.7	18.8	6.7	18.5	6.1	17.6	4.9	22.5	6.2	17.4	3.6	18.6	5.7
PCR	17.9	5.2	18.8	4.6	22.7	6.4	21.7	1.8	16.7	4.0	19.5	4.8	19.1	4.8
TCR	16.3	3.7	16.1	4.7	18.2	4.9	19.3	1.5	13.0	3.0	17.7	4.1	16.5	4.3
ILC	14.9	4.9	15.6	4.9	18.3	3.4	14.9	5.1	14.5	5.2	19.8	3.9	16.3	4.9
ERP	22.0	3.4	19.8	5.8	19.3	4.8	18.9	6.3	23.6	3.5	18.1	6.2	20.0	5.5

Tab. 9: IPQ part II mean scores stratified by illness group (Source: Own data)

Divergent validity and correlation with physical and mental health

Spearman correlation coefficients were calculated between the PANAS and the IPQ part II scale measures in order to make sure that the illness perceptions of patients do not merely reflect affective dispositions.

	TLA	TLC	CSQ	PCR	TCR	ILC	ERP
PA	-0.02	-0.05	-0.08	0.02	-0.14	0.15	0.00
NA	0.01	0.09	0.21	-0.14	-0.29*	-0.08	0.45*
PCS	-0.15	-0.43*	-0.34*	0.07	0.15	0.11	-0.39*
MCS	-0.26	-0.25	-0.45*	0.02	0.29*	0.22	-0.48*
SPHS[+]	0.10	0.14	0.22	-0.14	-0.13	-0.11	0.30*

Note. [+]The first item of the SF-12 was used as a measure of self-perceived health status; * p<0.05

Tab. 10: Correlations between IPQ part II and PANAS positive and negative affect measures as well as health indices (Source: Own data)

Tab. 10 shows that correlations were quite small with illness beliefs being slightly stronger correlated with negative than with positive affect. The strongest correlation could be identified between negative affect and emotional representation suggesting that about 20% of variance in the emotional reaction caused by the illness is accounted for by trait negative affect. While also treatment control was associated with trait NA, timeline, personal control, illness coherence, and consequences were not. No significant association existed between part II dimensions and positive affect. However, PCR and TCR had correlations of -0.14 and -0.15 respectively.

Several dimensions were associated with one or both measure of health-related quality of life. Also, self-perceived health status (SPHS) was associated negatively with emotional representations. Other associations were not significant.

IPQ-R part III

Part III of the IPQ-R on causal attribution was examined in the same way as part II, since it is identical as regards its underlying item format.

Structural validity and scale distribution

As with part II, several causal attributions were moderately correlated with each other. Significant coefficients ranged from 0.24 to 0.63. No strong correlation was identified (Tab. A 5). Likewise, PCA was used to examine the factor structure of the 19 items involved in part III of the IPQ-R.

The anti-image correlation matrix of these items shows that the proportion of items not shared by other items used for the PCA was lower than for part II of the IPQ, reflected by a Kaiser-Meyer-Olkin-Coefficient of 0.62. Accordingly, the anti-image correlation matrix shows that the proportion of high partial correlation coefficients was lower than in part II, as indicated by the values off the diagonal (Tab. A 6). Also, only five variables had an MSA slightly smaller than 0.5. These were the causal attributions "heredity", "microbes/virus", "diet", "smoking/alcohol", "God's will", and "nazar". According to their MSA, these would be candidate variables for exclusion from the model. However, in the first model, they were retained to replicate the solution found in the original and Turkish version. Bartlett's test of sphericity was highly significant (p<0.001). Pre-setting the number of factors to 4 that were identified in the original IPQ-R and its cultural adaptations, revealed the following factor solution (Tab. 11):

IPQ-R part III item	Factor 1	2	3	4	r_{itc}	α if deleted
Psychological attributions (PSY-CA), n=80, α=0.74						
D10: Family problems	.76	.25	.01	.13	.67	.65
D1: Stress or worry	.64	-.01	-.27	.15	.51	.70
D9: My mental attitude, e.g. thinking about life negatively	.57	.26	-.02	.18	.48	.71
D17: My personality	.32	.22	.46	.25	.30	.75
D12: My emotional state, e.g. feeling down lonely, anxious, empty	.73	.04	-.22	-.14	.48	.71
D11: Overwork	.65	.08	.10	.10	.46	.71
Risk factor attributions (RF-CA), n=81, α=0.48						
D15: Smoking or Alcohol	.00	.00	-.03	.77	.22	.45
D8: My own behavior	.34	.51	-.14	.28	.40	.35
D13: Aging	.51	-.11	.05	.43	.29	.40
D6: Poor medical care in the past	.51	.56	.32	-.05	.12	.49
D4: Diet or eating habits	.16	.14	-.63	.16	.33	.38
D2: Heredity	.10	.08	-.62	.10	.13	.50
Immune attributions (IMM-CA), n=77; α=0.33						
D18: Altered immunity	.65	-.10	.11	.01	.07	.55
D3: A germ or a virus	-.01	.79	-.14	.04	.18	.27
D7: Pollution in the environment	.26	.53	-.15	.49	.36	-.14
Chance/accident attributions (CHA-CA), n=78, α=0.45						
D16: Accident or injury	.06	.32	.49	.51	.25	.38
D5: Chance or bad luck	.45	.34	.26	-.28	.24	.39
D14: God's will	.30	-.43	.09	.28	.21	.42
D19: Nazar	.10	-.09	.57	.12	.31	.31

Tab. 11: Principal component analysis of IPQ-R part III items with original factor structure, rotated solution (Source: Own data)

Aside from the first factor whose items loaded pretty well (except "D17: My personality"), items in other dimensions had very poor loadings on their respective factors. This went together with poor internal consistencies in these three dimensions ranging from α=0.35 to α=0.48. Also, many items had very low inter-item correlations affecting scale homogeneities considerably. Furthermore, although no extremely low communalities of $h^2 < 0.10$ existed, average communality was $\bar{x} = 0.51$ ($s = 0.10$), ranging from 0.35 to 0.66 (not shown). Indeed, the solution outlined above made it hardly possible to identify the factor structure extracted in the original version of the IPQ-R (and replicated by the Turkish validation). Because part II of the IPQ-R is based on the theoretical framework developed by Leventhal and each of the seven dimensions represents one of the SRM's core components, it did not make sense to find an alternative factor solution for this IPQ-R section. However, this is different for part III where no framework exists. Hence, the measures mentioned previously can be applied to find a better factor solution and to increase scale internal consistency and homogeneity. This is especially important considering the performance of the structure shown in Tab. 11 that, except for factor 1, does not allow deriving any practical use of the extracted dimensions.

With a KMO of 0.62 the overall sample adequacy was not optimal. It was negatively affected by several variables as indicated by their low MSAs smaller than 0.50 (see Tab. A 6). For an alternative model, the variables "D2: Heredity", "D4: Diet or eating habits", and "D15: Smoking or Alcohol" that all had MSAs<0.5 have been excluded from analysis to improve overall sample adequacy. Although also "D3: A germ or a virus", "D14: God's will", and "D19: Nazar" had suboptimal sample adequacies, D2 and D4 have been given preference for exclusion over D3, D14, and D19, because, on theoretical grounds, they describe a dimension (i.e. risk factor attribution) that is also represented by a sufficient number of other variables. This is neither the case for D14 and D19 nor for D3. Excluding these variables would have not allowed extracting the factor "Chance/accident attributions" and "Immune attributions" that only consist of four and three variables, respectively. By excluding D2, D4, and D15, KMO could be increased to a value of 0.70 reaching a mediocre level.

As described in the methods section, different extraction criteria have been applied to identify an improved solution for part III of the IPQ-R. However, these criteria—a situation quite typical for factor analysis—each suggested a different number of factors to be extracted (see visualization in Fig. 10). The Kaiser's eigenvalue criterion >1 suggested a five-factor solution accounting for about 63.2% of cumulative variance and producing factors with a little number of items and many cross-loadings. Basing the number of factors to be extracted on the graphic visualization of a scree plot that plots the number of factors against their corresponding eigenvalues, two, three or six factors were to be extracted. The two-factor solution had an average h^2 of 0.38 ($s = 0.16$) and explained 38.8% of cumulative variance. Factors, however, were difficult to interpret, because many cross-loadings existed and items had positive and negative loadings where equally directed loadings would have been expected. Same as the five-factor solution, the six-factor solution was not practical because dimensions with few items had been created. While the original and revised minimum average partial test (MAP) both suggest a one factor solution, three factors are to be extracted following the parallel analysis for PCA. Here, the 95%-percentile of the random eigenvalue distribution on the basis of 1000 samples with 82 cases and 16 variables for the first five components is 1.86, 1.65, 1.50, 1.38, and 1.27. The observed eigenvalue distribution for the first five factors in the current sample is 4.54, 1.66, 1.60, 1.27, and 1.09. Following the instruction for parallel analysis, those factors had to be extracted whose observed eigenvalues were above the random eigenvalue distribution. In the present case, this was true for the first three factors (see Fig. 10). By suggesting three factors, parallel analysis identified the same number of factors as had been identified on the basis of the scree plot. These three factors accounted for 38.8% of shared variance.

IPQ-R part III item	Factor 1	2	3	r_{itc}	α if de- leted
Physical/psychological attributions ($PHY-CA), n=81, α=0.80					
D10: Family problems	.73	.26	.23	.68	.74
D1: Stress or worry	.73	.14	-.18	.54	.77
D11: Overwork	.67	.18	.06	.54	.77
D12: My emotional state, e.g. feeling down lonely, anxious, empty	.67	-.02	.12	.50	.78
D18: Altered immunity	.65	-.06	.09	.48	.78
D13: Aging	.55	-.01	.19	.46	.78
D9: My mental attitude, e.g. thinking about life negatively	.55	.28	.21	.48	.78
Risk factor/environmental attributions ($RFE-CA), n=77, α=0.68					
D3: A germ or a virus	-.06	.77	.11	.43	.63
D7: Pollution in the environment	.34	.69	.01	.54	.56
D8: My own behavior	.31	.52	.24	.43	.63
D6: Poor medical care in the past	.39	.49	.41	.45	.62
Chance/accident attributions ($CHA-CA), n=78, α=0.52					
D14: God's will	.28	-.46	.34	.18	.54
D16: Accident or injury	-.03	.26	.69	.37	.43
D19: Nazar	-.04	-.26	.64	.34	.44
D17: My personality	.20	.12	.63	.33	.45
D5: Chance or bad luck	.25	.14	.50	.27	.48

Tab. 12: Principal component analysis of IPQ-R part III items with revised factor structure, ro- tated solution (Source: Own data)

The revised three-factor structure illustrated in Tab. 12 has several improvements over the original four factor solution: First, factor loadings are considerably higher and cross-loadings considerably lower than in the original structure, making it possi- ble to identify three distinct factors. This also becomes evident when these factors are plotted against each other (not shown). The three factors are separated from one another with only D3 and D14 moderately loading on the third factor. Also, no re- versed loadings in primary factors exist. Second, internal consistency of the three scales is higher than it was for the four-factor solution. It is α=0.80 for the first, α=0.68 for the second, and α=0.52 for the third factor. Only two items have corrected item-total correlations of less than 0.30. Third, saturation of items per factor is higher than in the original solution, since no factor has three or fewer items which could be considered problematic in terms of reliability. Following the dimension labels of the original structure, the three factors can be labeled as "Physical/psychological attribu- tions", "Risk factor/environmental attributions", and "Chance/accident attributions". The last factor, "chance/accident attributions", is still not optimal as reflected by the low r_{itc}'s and a comparably low internal consistency. Most probably, the revised factor solution could be further improved by deleting the variables 'D14: God's will' and 'D19: Nazar' that performed sub-optimally regarding their sample adequacy (MSAs<0.5). However, for theoretical reasons, they were retained in the model in order to sufficiently account for the role of supernatural causal attributions.

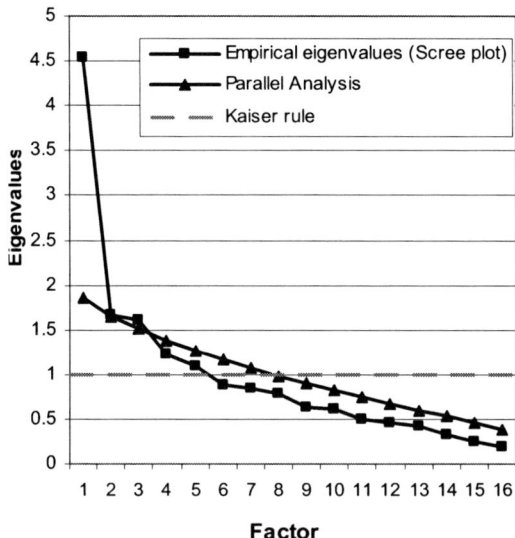

Fig. 10: Scree plot and parallel analysis of IPQ-R part III items (alternative solution)
(Source: Own data)

Because the original factor structure does not allow forming any meaningful scales or scores, all following summary measures for the part III dimensions are based on the revised factor structure (denoted by $ in abbreviations). Since there is no underlying theoretical framework for this section of the IPQ-R, proceeding like this makes sense for exploratory purposes. Factor scores were computed and missing values substituted in the same way as was described for the original factor structure except that items were attributed to factors on the basis of the revised solution.

Fig. A 2 shows the distribution of the newly computed factor scores over the entire sample. The physical/psychological attributions score ($PHY-CA) and the chance/accident attributions score ($CHA-CA) resemble normal distributions as is also supported by the non-significant Shapiro-Wilks-test.

	Diabetes		Cardio-vasc.		Respiratory		Cancer		Mental		Other		Total	
	x̄	s	x̄	s	x̄	s	x̄	s	x̄	s	x̄	s	x̄	s
$PHY-CA	20.2	6.4	20.9	7.4	21.0	8.6	21.3	6.2	21.1	8.3	16.8	7.2	20.1	7.3
$RFE-CA	9.3	4.4	9.0	3.0	10.2	2.8	7.6	3.4	11.0	4.9	9.9	4.1	9.3	3.6
$CHA-CA	12.3	4.2	13.1	3.3	12.5	2.3	12.9	4.7	14.4	6.6	9.8	5.0	12.4	4.4

Tab. 13: Causal attributions (IPQ-R part III) mean scores stratified by illness group
(Source: Own data)

Means and standard deviations stratified by illness groups are illustrated in Tab. 13. Scores are similar among the different groups. Patients categorized into the illness group "other physical diseases" had slightly lower beliefs in all three dimensions. No significant differences between illness groups could be identified when controlling for multiple comparisons.

Divergent validity

To assess divergent validity, causal attributions were correlated with the positive and negative affect measures.

	$PSY-CA	$RFE-CA	$CHA-CA
PA	0.09	0.20*	0.24*
NA	-0.29*	-0.11	-0.02

Note. * p<0.05

Tab. 14: Correlations between IPQ-R part III scales and PANAS positive and negative affect measures (Source: Own data)

Tab. 14 illustrates that correlations are quite small with attributions being weakly correlated with both affects. The three strongest associations were identified between psychological attributions (r_s=-0.29) and negative affect as well as between positive affect and chance attributions (r_s=-0.24) and risk factor/environmental attributions (r_s=0.20), with the other causes showing the same tendency.

Correlations between IPQ-R dimensions

Spearman correlation coefficients were calculated to examine the relationship between IPQ-R dimensions (Tab. A 7). The two timeline dimensions correlated most strongly with perceived consequences of a disease and, as regards chronic timeline, with emotional representations. Emotional representations were also correlated with perceived consequences and illness coherence. Furthermore, several core beliefs were associated with causal attributions. While illness coherence showed a significant positive association with physical/psychological attributions and positive but insignificant associations with the other attributions, other beliefs were associated negatively with causal attributions, of which only timeline chronic, consequences, and emotional representations were correlated significantly. Causal attributions were also positively correlated with one another.

The Brief IPQ

Scale distribution

Fig. A 3 gives an overview of the item distribution of the Brief IPQ. None of the items had a normal distribution. Instead, most items were skewed to the right.

Item means varied across illness groups. On average, individuals with mental diseases had higher scores than the other groups, however no statistically significant differences were identified (Tab. 15).

	Diabetes		Cardio-vasc.		Respiratory		Cancer		Mental		Other		Total	
	$\bar{x}$	s	$\bar{x}$	s	$\bar{x}$	s	$\bar{x}$	s	$\bar{x}$	s	$\bar{x}$	s	$\bar{x}$	s
G1: Consequ.	7.50	2.71	6.70	2.95	7.00	2.76	5.14	3.76	9.00	1.77	5.88	2.80	6.77	2.94
G2: Timeline	8.67	2.19	6.87	3.05	8.83	2.04	5.43	3.21	8.00	2.78	8.25	1.84	7.56	2.75
G3: Pers.Contr.	6.27	2.65	5.06	3.55	5.50	2.35	5.57	3.99	6.75	3.49	6.25	2.46	5.72	3.16
G4: Treat.Contr.	6.00	2.00	7.06	2.63	6.80	1.79	7.50	1.52	5.63	3.54	6.75	2.11	6.71	2.43
G5: Identity	7.92	2.39	6.97	2.41	6.80	2.77	5.71	3.68	7.88	3.36	5.75	2.49	6.83	2.71
G6: Concern	8.42	1.78	7.23	2.73	6.60	2.30	5.57	3.95	8.88	1.64	5.75	2.79	7.09	2.78
G7: Coherence	6.00	3.07	6.61	3.34	8.20	1.92	7.71	3.55	5.13	4.70	6.63	2.75	6.57	3.28
G8: Emotions	7.75	2.34	6.56	2.99	5.60	3.36	5.86	3.72	8.63	2.67	5.75	3.40	6.66	3.10

Tab. 15: Brief IPQ item mean scores stratified by illness group (Source: Own data)

Convergent validity

To assess the convergent validity of the Brief IPQ, correlation coefficients (Spearman r_s) between the dimensions of the Brief IPQ and the IPQ-R were calculated. As shown in Tab. 16, most IPQ-R part II dimensions and their 11-point single item counterparts from the Brief IPQ were correlated. IPQ-R personal and treatment control scales and the corresponding scales of the Brief IPQ, however, were not correlated. IPQ-R emotional representations were associated with the Brief IPQ consequences, concerns, identity, and emotions scale.

	G1: Con-sequences	G2: Timeline	G3: Personal control	G4: Treatment control	G5: Identity	G6: Concern	G7:Coherence/Comprehension	G8: Emotions
TLA	0.23*	0.23	-0.05	-0.06	0.09	0.10	-0.02	-0.03
TLC	0.29*	-0.06	-0.04	-0.12	0.33*	0.26*	0.03	0.06
CSQ	0.31*	0.18	-0.15	-0.25*	0.23*	0.18	-0.01	0.20
PCR	-0.09	-0.01	-0.21	-0.16	-0.09	-0.12	0.12	-0.17
TCR	-0.26*	-0.22	-0.05	0.12	-0.15	-0.17	0.05	-0.33*
ILC	-0.08	0.14	0.06	-0.11	-0.16	-0.24*	0.27*	-0.20
ERP	0.56*	0.12	0.09	-0.09	0.42*	0.50*	-0.06	0.40*
$PSY-CA	0.35*	-0.04	0.06	0.11	0.42*	0.31*	-0.01	0.32*
$RFE-CA	0.05	0.06	0.00	-0.09	0.26*	-0.01	0.01	0.08
$CHA-CA	0.15	-0.15	0.02	-0.18	0.11	0.06	0.03	0.05

Note. *p<0.05

Tab. 16: Correlation matrix of Brief IPQ and IPQ-R part II dimensions (Source: Own data)

Unlike the IPQ-R that applies a multiple item battery to examine causal attributions, the Brief IPQ utilizes an open-ended question to assess beliefs about causes of illness. In order to determine its validity, responses given to this question were compared with part III of the IPQ-R. Tab. 17 presents the four top-rated causes as measured by the IPQ-R.

	Diabetes	Cardiovas-cular disease	Respiratory Disease	Cancer	Mental condi-tions
1.	- God's will	- God's will	- Altered immunity	- Altered immunity	- Chance or fate
2.	- Aging	- Stress	- God's will	- Stress	- God's will
3.	- Heredity	- Aging	- Mental attitude	- God's will	- Heredity
4.	- Family problems/ overwork/emo-tional state*	- Over work	- Aging	- Overwork	- Poor past medical care

Note. Rating is based on the median of each item; *all three causes rated equally

Tab. 17: The four top-rated causes as measured by part III of the IPQ-R (Source: Own data)

With one exception, these causes were also the most frequently endorsed factors on the qualitative item of the Brief IPQ. Although "God's will" was rated very highly on the IPQ-R, it was almost non-existent in responses to the open-ended question of the Brief IPQ. Of all causes given in response to this qualitative item, most (80.7%) could be categorized within the 19 causal factors of the IPQ-R. Additional causes mentioned sporadically by patients and not part of the IPQ-R were for example psychological factors like yearning, sorrow and sadness, physical conditions like illnesses and pain, and environmental factors like problems at work and language barriers.

Divergent validity

As with the two IPQ-R sections, Spearman correlation coefficients between the Brief IPQ items and the two PANAS affect scales were calculated to make sure that illness perceptions of patients did not merely reflect affective dispositions.

	G1: Con-sequences	G2: Timeline	G3: Per-sonal con-trol	G4: Treat-ment control	G5: Identity	G6: Concern	G7: Coher-ence/Com-prehension	G8: Emotions
PA	0.09	0.11	0.15	0.12	-0.01	0.08	-0.08	0.05
NA	0.33*	0.13	0.11	-0.12	0.32*	0.34*	-0.27*	0.30*
PCS	-0.46*	-0.18	0.18	0.21	-0.43*	-0.42*	0.10	-0.28*
MCS	-0.53*	-0.17	-0.03	0.03	-0.32*	-0.46*	0.07	-0.40*
SPHS	0.27*	-0.06	0.05	-0.04	0.17	0.22	-0.07	0.11

Note. * p<0.05

Tab. 18: Correlations between Brief IPQ items and positive and negative affect measures as well as health indices (Source: Own data)

Tab. 18 shows that the divergent validity of the Brief IPQ resembles that of the IPQ-R (see Tab. 10), since the correlation matrices were similar to each other. The strongest correlation could be identified between negative affect and concern followed by negative affect and emotional representations and negative affect and identity. As was the case for part II of the IPQ-R, no significant association could be identified between positive affect and Brief IPQ dimensions. Several dimensions were associated with one or both measures of HRQOL. Self-rated health was only associated with perceived consequences of a disease.

4.2.3 The usability of the IPQ-R and the Brief IPQ

In total, 58 persons participated in the qualitative survey, 70% of which were women. Although interview questions were open-ended and asked by the interviewers in a way to stimulate participants' motivation to talk, responses and comments were very short, not very detailed, and mostly very positive. According to the responses, almost all patients had a very positive impression about the questionnaire and its language (91.7%), had neither difficulties in understanding questions, wordings, or single expressions nor identified ambiguous words (90.0%), and found that the questionnaire overall was very clear and comprehensible (88.3%). Of these, some mentioned they had liked it to write down what they are thinking or how they experience their illness and treatment (10.0%). Others were happy about the research interest and that the study was carried out in Turkish language:

- *"I was very happy about the survey on my illness. I am very satisfied with it!"* (Male patient, 57 years old, lives in Germany for 22 years; questionnaire interviewer-administered);

- *"I liked the questionnaire and its style, because it is my own language"* (Male patient, 65 years old, lives in Germany for 15 years, questionnaire self-administered);

- *"Very good. Our language"* (Male patient, 71 years old, lives in Germany for 35 years, questionnaire self-administered);

- *"The questionnaire was well prepared"* (Female patient, 46 years old, lives in Germany for 23 years, questionnaire interviewer-administered).

Very few patients mentioned that they did not fully understand all questions and that sometimes words and phrases were complicated, ambiguous, or misleading. However, in interviews with these patients, it was not possible to identify those misleading expressions. Others mentioned they would not have understood everything if it had not been read and explained to them in different words.

Although the number of interviewees with a positive critique of the questionnaire was very high, it has to be questioned whether the overall understanding and usability of the questionnaire was really as good as the results of the qualitative survey suggest. The reason for this doubt is the discrepancy to impressions the research team gained during the quantitative survey. Here, it became clear more frequently than in the qualitative survey that patients had problems with item wordings, phrases, and expressions. Interviewer-administered and assisted self-administered surveys showed that patients encountered most problems with the SF-12 whose language was obviously experienced as too intellectual and too scientific resulting in lower comprehensibility of the instrument. In the course of the surveys, some respondents as well as other Turkish speaking persons involved in the surveys (e.g. clinic personnel) pointed at some easier wordings and expressions those currently used in the SF-12 could be replaced with. A possible revision of the SF-12 will be discussed in chapter 5.1.2.

While the difficulties patients encountered with the SF-12 were due to language style, conceptual issues emerged with the identity scale. As is also reflected by the very high number of missing values, patients had substantial problems with correctly understanding the two subscales (left- and right-hand side) of the identity scale. During the surveys, many had stated they did not see any difference between both scales—despite a straight forward wording and additional highlighting (*"I have experienced this symptom since the beginning of my illness"* vs. *"This symptom is related to my disease"*). Additionally, respondents complained about the similarity of a number of items in part II of the IPQ-R (*"I filled that already in just now"* being one statement frequently made) referring to the similarly of the wording used in each dimension that only offers subtle nuances.

Patients encountered different problems with filling in part II items. Difficulties in understanding in particular regarded items C2, C10, C14, C33, and C34. Some patients also requested examples for items C12, C13, and C15. In contrast to the experiences gained during the pre-test, most participants had no difficulty in filling in the Brief IPQ. Although very few (3.8%) said the scale was misleading and they did not understand how to interpret the numbers between the two end-points, others mentioned it should be clear to everybody when reading the explanation in the introductory part. In case the instrument would be subject to revision, some participants said it could be considered changing the response format by labeling the response categories and reducing the number of response levels, thus making it similar to part II and III of the IPQ-R.

A conceptual problem also emerged with question 7 asking patients about their disease. Usually, the IPQ-R is tailored to patients' diseases, which means that it is usually not necessary for patients to give information about their disease state. Hence, the disease patients suffer from is known beforehand and is not based on patient self-report as was the case in the current study. Aside from the possible discrepancies between self-report and objective information, some patients sometimes quoted more than one illness despite the instruction to quote only the one with the longest history of medical treatment. Especially, they often ticked one of the four major illnesses (diabetes, cardiovascular disease, renal disease, asthma) and additionally quoted another conditions under the response category "other". These misunderstandings could be immediately resolved, since respondents brought up their confusion during the survey.

While most patients were happy that their native language was used in the questionnaire, 5 patients were complaining that no German version was available. Although local coordinators indicated the proficiency in Turkish and German language for each patient and although only those participants whose primary language was Turkish, these few persons had been misclassified (not shown in Fig. 5). In all 5 cases, their proficiency in German was higher than that in Turkish resulting in lower comprehensibility of the questionnaire and frustration (*"You should better give me a German version of this. This way, I would be better able to get through with it"*, *Female patient, 40 years old*). Of these 5 patients, 2 were not willing to complete, because they feared their responses would not be anonymous and wondered why it were only people with Turkish background who were the target group of the survey and not other groups. Responses from the remaining 3 patients were excluded from analysis.

Due to the questionnaire length, test-taker burden was not low. Patients who were able to fill in questionnaires themselves needed 20 to 35 minutes for completion, while interviewer-administered questionnaires took slightly longer (30 to 45 minutes).

4.3   What do the empirical findings mean?

Research has shown that by attaching greater importance to the diversity of illness perceptions in the health care process, patients' coping strategies and treatment outcomes can be improved. This study prepared the ground for the quantitative assessment of illness perceptions in a population that, due to its culture, its tradition, its norm, its value systems, and its social situation may be different from the German population in terms of this important psychological construct.

We applied the IPQ-R and the Brief IPQ—two instruments that have shown good psychometric properties in English speaking countries—to Turkish migrants residing in Germany. While a version of the IPQ-R validated among Turks residing in Turkey existed, this study identified starting points for a further adaptation of the same instrument for persons with a Turkish migration background in Germany. Also, by translating and testing the Brief IPQ, it made a well-established short version of the powerful IPQ-R applicable to Turkish language communities, enhancing the practical use of an instrument utilizing a rich framework for the assessment of illness perceptions.

Knowledge about the illness perceptions of Turkish migrants gained by a properly adapted Turkish migrant version of the IPQ-R and the Brief IPQ could be used to tailor health care services to the needs of migrants and to intervene into their coping strategies by means of counseling services targeting the modification of beliefs disadvantageous for optimal coping. The valid and reliable assessment of illness perceptions in migrants, hence, can be considered an essential part of culture- and migrant-specific health care. This study showed that the IPQ-R and the Brief IPQ have the potential to serve this purpose. However, first different obstacles need to be considered and tackled.

4.3.1 IPQ-R part I

Due to a large number of missing values, the lowest performance as regards validity was shown by part I of the IPQ-R. Although it is straight forward, demands less concentration from the respondent, is quite fast and easy to fill in, and thus has a lower amount of test-taker burden as compared to the other parts of the IPQ-R, it caused difficulties when administered. While missings for the left-hand side of the IPQ-part I ranged from 6.1 to 19.5%, up to half of all respondents did not fill in the right-hand side of the instrument. Most of the other half gave responses identical to the left-hand side. While the fact that these responses are the same between both subscales could theoretically be a true effect due to lack of differences between illness somatization and identity (cf. Moss-Morris et al. 2002), considering the missing values and the statements made during the survey, this phenomenon is rather more likely to be due to a misunderstanding. Obviously, the differences between both subscales of the identity scale were not clear to the participants, resulting in a misinterpretation of the

IPQ-R part I. This was neither the case in the original nor in the Turkish adaptation (no validations of part I exist for other language adaptations). Additional or modified instructions should be included in future versions to ensure the understanding of this IPQ-R section by Turkish migrants.

4.3.2 IPQ-R part II

As regards the *structural validity* of the IPQ-R part II, potential for improvement could be identified. Tab. 19 compares the factor structures generated in the current study to the factor structures of the original IPQ-R, the Italian version by Giardini et al. (2007), and the Turkish translation by Kocaman et al. (2007) by means of factor loadings and internal consistencies as determined by Cronbach's α.

Factor	Current study							Italian (Giardini et al. 2007)							Original (Moss-Morris et al. 2002)							TR*
	1	2	3	4	5	6	7	1	2	3	4	5	6	7	1	2	3	4	5	6	7	
TLA	α=.57							α=.76							α=.89							α=.72
C1	-.01	.40	-.31	-.15	-.03	.30	.17	-.04	.01	-.04	-.14	.52	.10	.37	.05	.07	-.04	-.15	.76	-.01	.08	.41
C2	-.04	-.07	.02	.04	.82	-.11	.07	.14	.07	.06	-.02	.66	.04	-.10	.08	.07	-.13	-.05	.83	.02	.12	.53
C3	.00	.03	-.10	.15	.85	-.03	.03	.04	.16	.02	-.06	.83	-.07	-.01	.05	.07	-.13	-.10	.86	.02	.13	.59
C4	.14	.36	-.47	.12	.35	.12	.16	-.03	-.03	-.01	-.10	.53	.00	.31	.12	-.07	-.07	-.13	.75	-.09	.16	.51
C5	.11	.14	.27	-.17	.56	.06	.37	.00	.16	-.08	.07	.76	.01	.11	.01	.10	-.07	-.10	.82	.02	.20	.52
C18	.06	.13	-.17	-.57	.19	.37	-.26	-.02	.26	-.30	-.46	.39	.13	.21	-.08	.01	-.20	-.44	.61	.09	.14	.47
TLC	α=.36							α=.73							α=.79							α=.71
C29	.57	.14	.25	.17	-.04	-.08	.12	.09	.73	-.03	.04	.17	-.17	.20	.08	.71	-.11	.03	.01	.11	.13	.49
C30	.09	-.26	.42	.01	.27	-.11	-.01	.01	.78	-.10	.14	.04	.11	.12	.01	.84	.06	.07	.03	-.08	-.04	.42
C31	.36	-.36	.06	-.09	-.06	-.12	-.23	.15	.61	-.18	-.10	.15	.01	-.14	.08	.72	-.06	-.13	.07	.25	.07	.38
C32	.62	.20	.18	-.12	.24	.23	-.02	.22	.60	-.07	.07	.17	-.09	-.10	.15	.73	-.09	-.02	.08	-.02	.01	.49
CSQ	α=.71							α=.64							α=.84							α=.69
C6	.08	.11	.38	-.31	.40	.05	.35	.27	.19	.03	.10	.60	.10	-.29	.09	.09	-.01	-.04	.49	.01	.57	.57
C7	.43	.44	.30	-.23	.38	-.02	.16	.35	.18	.08	.17	.58	.04	-.09	.16	.05	-.02	-.12	.38	.04	.74	.59
C8	.16	.59	.14	-.18	.24	-.17	-.10	.16	.08	.23	-.02	.10	.21	.54	.23	.05	-.05	-.32	.13	-.06	.55	.33
C9	.39	-.24	-.15	-.02	.23	.10	.48	.51	.31	.17	-.04	.21	.01	-.03	.14	.01	-.17	-.13	.03	.14	.73	.48
C10	.26	-.06	.04	-.01	.10	.03	.75	.28	.34	-.05	-.06	.38	.01	-.10	.25	.13	-.11	-.05	.24	.10	.67	.48
C11	.36	.00	.16	.00	.14	-.25	.75	.25	.44	.16	-.02	.10	.06	-.01	.30	-.04	-.07	-.15	.12	.08	.70	.58
PCR	α=.59							α=.50							α=.81							α=.70
C12	-.01	-.07	.68	.17	-.04	.18	.17	-.09	.05	.17	.58	.05	-.07	.09	-.13	.14	.51	.50	.01	-.08	-.15	.48
C13	.06	.33	.66	.18	.13	.04	.05	.08	.02	.19	.46	.28	.02	-.28	-.06	-.01	.56	.42	-.18	-.11	-.06	.49
C14	-.14	-.02	.81	.15	-.01	-.10	-.09	-.12	.08	.14	.59	-.06	.04	-.35	-.14	-.02	.51	.50	-.21	.01	-.14	.59
C15	-.10	.80	.05	.18	-.02	.17	-.07	-.03	-.16	.75	-.01	.05	.04	.29	-.03	-.03	.76	.10	-.11	-.10	-.02	.47
C16	.16	-.42	.49	.24	.04	.22	.20	.00	-.13	.00	.48	.03	.12	-.22	-.15	-.05	.57	.38	-.13	-.11	.03	.51
C17	-.03	.56	-.07	-.10	.03	.19	-.01	-.09	-.02	.71	-.02	-.04	.20	-.09	-.03	-.08	.73	.08	-.07	-.16	-.12	.36
TCR	α=.70							α=.59							α=.80							α=.75
C19	-.08	.51	-.15	.33	-.33	.01	-.10	-.21	-.19	.38	.22	-.41	.12	.00	-.15	-.12	.30	.56	-.26	-.16	-.11	.34
C20	.14	-.10	.31	.67	.05	.08	.17	-.13	.02	-.22	.61	-.19	.10	-.03	.04	-.03	-.10	.61	-.53	.04	-.05	.66
C21	-.13	.02	.08	.82	.04	.03	-.08	-.02	.18	-.03	.68	.01	.05	.08	-.03	.02	.13	.79	-.12	-.07	-.19	.65
C22	.15	.17	.23	.69	.24	.16	-.23	.05	-.08	-.30	.67	-.09	.11	.27	-.05	.04	.19	.81	-.07	-.08	-.14	.47
C23	-.24	.49	-.09	.47	-.14	.05	-.16	-.22	-.14	.21	.21	-.14	.54	-.20	-.08	-.13	.35	.58	-.22	-.18	-.08	.34
ILC	α=.72							α=.73							α=.87							α=.73
C24	-.56	.11	.10	.01	.02	.39	-.06	-.47	-.27	.07	.09	-.18	.35	-.02	.17	.24	-.09	.10	.02	.73	.19	.31
C25	-.06	.13	-.04	-.17	-.15	.72	.07	-.30	-.05	.03	.02	.01	.72	.19	.15	.05	-.13	.01	.02	.86	.10	.38
C26	-.20	.11	.04	.15	-.07	.78	-.06	-.20	-.04	.02	.00	.00	.81	.15	.13	.04	-.12	-.14	-.04	.86	.06	.43
C27	-.34	.37	-.10	.13	-.04	.59	.03	-.06	-.14	.10	.08	.06	.69	.05	.16	.09	-.18	-.10	.01	.83	.13	.37
C28	.14	-.17	.26	.17	.28	.55	-.19	.02	.03	-.06	.13	.20	.50	-.31	.18	-.03	-.18	-.14	-.01	.64	-.16	.52

Factor	Current study							Italian (Giardini et al. 2007)							Original (Moss-Morris et al. 2002)							TR*
	1	2	3	4	5	6	7	1	2	3	4	5	6	7	1	2	3	4	5	6	7	
ERP	α=.69							α=.82							α=.88							α=.77
C33	.80	-.05	.02	.01	.06	-.12	.05	.79	.15	.00	-.05	-.05	-.15	.11	.79	.07	-.16	-.03	.06	.12	.21	.68
C34	.83	-.01	-.12	-.02	.05	-.15	.08	.86	.01	-.05	-.03	.02	-.08	.13	.83	.01	-.18	.06	.03	.16	.22	.68
C35	.64	.00	-.17	.01	-.06	-.26	.28	.86	.09	-.05	.00	-.04	-.11	.10	.71	.10	-.13	-.01	-.02	.12	.25	.64
C36	-.41	.08	-.23	-.06	.12	.01	-.19	.29	.12	.16	-.19	.04	.34	.14	.61	.13	.11	-.22	-.03	.02	.20	.40
C37	.75	-.12	-.05	.01	.04	.05	.06	.70	.09	-.12	-.07	.18	-.12	-.13	.72	.00	.04	-.01	-.07	.18	.08	.61
C38	.69	-.10	-.05	-.14	.08	.06	.23	not shown due to misprint in publication							.70	.14	-.09	-.02	.16	.26	.03	.67

Note. * Turkish version by Kocaman et al. 2007 (since the authors only provide loadings for primary factors, results have been noted in a single column here).

Tab. 19: Comparison of the factor structures of the current study, the Italian, Original, and Turkish version by means of factor loading and consistency coefficients (Source: Own illustration)

Compared to the original version, the current factor structure has more cross-loadings. These, to a certain degree, may be due to chance considering the low sample size of n=82 in the current study. However, the "unclean" solution could also be the result of diverging concepts between the original and the current population as outlined above. If this was the case, a similar phenomenon should have occurred in Kocaman et al.'s (2007) sample. Unfortunately, it is not possible to test this assumption, since the authors did not provide factor loadings for other than the primary factor. In the present case, cross-loadings are problematic because in some cases they exceeded the primary loadings. While several cross-loadings above 0.40 (considered problematic according to literature on factor analysis; e.g. Hinton 2004) also existed in the original version, none of these exceeded the primary loadings. The Italian version, however, is similar to the current study with regard to high cross-loadings exceeding primary loadings, though to a slightly smaller extent. The considerably larger sample size of Giardini et al.'s (2007) sample (n=277) further suggests that not chance alone is responsible for this phenomenon.

Another difference between the four solutions concerns the size of the primary loadings that are all larger than 0.50 in the original version, ranging from 0.50 to 0.86. In the present population, primary loadings were lower, ranging from 0.05 to 0.82 (with two primary loadings being negative, -0.41 and -0.05). Eight primary loadings were below the threshold of |0.30| that indicates that an item is not suitable to form a factor (Bühner 2006). The Italian version, however, has even 12 items loading below |0.30|, five of which belong to the consequences scale making C8 the only item loading above 0.30. In the Italian and the current study, these "unclean" solutions are accompanied by lower internal consistencies as compared to the original version. Considering 0.65 or 0.70 as a sufficient consistency according to rules of thumb (Hinton 2004), the scales on emotional representations, illness coherence, treatment control, and consequences, in the present validation, perform well, while the scales on timeline acute and personal control remain slightly below the threshold. They could be improved by the deletion of item C1 ("My illness will last a short time") and C17 ("My actions will have no effect on the outcome of my illness") which would increase consistencies of the respective scales to α=0.61 and α=0.64, respectively (Tab. 8). These however, would still stay below the threshold making further improvement on the level prior to performing factor analysis necessary. The timeline cyclical scale performs worst because only one primary loading is above |0.30|—which is similar to the situation with the Italian consequences scale. Additionally, 2 of 4 primary loadings are negative although all items have been reversed correctly before analysis. Considering the higher loadings on the first factor (3 of 4 above |0.30| with no loading being negative), the choice of factor two does not seem appropriate. Instead, in an exploratory approach, when no factor structure would be known or set a priori, based on factor loadings, one would tend to attribute items C29, C31, C32 (and item C7 of the consequences scale) to the emotional representations scale. In all other versions displayed in the table above, the TLC scale discriminates well against the other factors. As the other discrepancies, this may be attributable to a number of possible reasons, among them chance and diverging populations and differences in concepts hold. Although the current adaptation performs less well as regards the TLC dimension that has the lowest internal consistency among all other factors, it performs better in the consequences scale and in the two control scales as compared to the Italian version.

Despite populations being considerably different between the four studies and conditions for factor analysis not being optimal in the current study, a similar pattern in all four factor structures can be identified. For example, in all studies, the emotional representations scale was among the ones performing best in comparison to the other factors. Furthermore, the first item of the treatment control scale had a high negative cross-loading on the timeline acute/chronic scale in all studies but Kocaman et al.'s. The last item of the timeline acute/chronic scale cross-loaded highly on the treatment control scale. The first two items of the consequences scale had high loadings on the timeline acute/chronic scale. In all non-original studies, the personal control scale had the lowest internal consistency. Also, the first item of the illness coherence scale had a high cross-loading on the timeline acute/chronic scale in both the current and the Italian study. On the one hand, these similarities reveal instrument immanent shortcomings. On the other hand, they might give support for the transferability of concepts and the applicability of the instrument to other cultures because similar phenomena occur in different populations. While some of these phenomena are still tolerable in the original version because primary loadings and internal consistencies are sufficiently high, they are susceptible to problems in populations other than the original. Due to lack of information, it is not possible to draw any conclusion regarding these phenomena in the study by Kocaman et al. (2007). Judged by the primary loadings and the internal consistencies alone, one can tell that factors performed better than either in the current or the Italian adaptation.

As the only study, Kocaman et al. (2007) also provided item-total correlations for all 38 items of part II (not shown in the table above). They reveal that item saturation is much higher than in the current study although no modifications as compared to the original study have been performed. C15 ("Nothing I do will affect my illness") and C36 ("My illness does not worry me") are the only items in the Turkish validation study having item-total correlation coefficients below 0.30, which can be considered the threshold for a sufficient saturation (cf. Bühner 2006). In the current study, C15 and C36 also perform poorly regarding their r_{itc}'s. However, there are also other items with r_{itc}'s<0.30, especially in the TLC scale that has already been outlined as problematic and of little practical use considering its poor psychometric properties. Item

C36 is the only item with a negative total-item correlation and the only item of the ERP scale with a negative factor loading. Since all reversed items have been recoded prior to analysis, this may go back to a misunderstanding due to the preceding seven and the last two items representing negative statements. This could be the consequence of Turkish grammar using agglutination, i.e. the joining of affixes to word roots to form expressions. Hence, *"Hastalığım beni endişelendirmiyor" ("My illness does not worry me")* could have easily been confused with *"Hastalığım beni endişelendiriyor" ("My illness does worry me")*. This aspect will be further discussed below.

Taking the "unclean" solutions of the current and the Italian studies with their partially low primary loadings and low internal consistencies into consideration, it is surprising that Kocaman et al. (2007) achieved results comparable to the original version. In fact, the results of the factor solution of the present study are more comparable to the Italian solution than they are to the Turkish study. It is difficult to find an explanation for why part II of the instrument in that study, without any tweaks, performed as good as the original, while the present and the Italian study revealed a lower validity of the instrument in their respective populations. However, it has to be mentioned that Kocaman et al. (2007) administered the questionnaire to their participants by means of interviews, while the Italian study solely relied on self-administration and the current study used a dual mixed-mode assessment depending on the preference of the individuals.

In the current study, the factor results of part II clearly suggest tweaking the factor model to obtain more stable results. This would involve selecting a set of the 38 items based on the anti-correlation matrix and the extraction of differently composed factors. This procedure was chosen in the two Spanish versions (Marcos et al. 2005; Vázquez et al. 2007) resulting in the elimination of several items and five- and six-factor solutions, respectively. As can be seen in the factor matrix that is provided by Vázquez et al. (2007), factors discriminated well against one another because cross-loadings were negligible, primary loadings were high ranging from +/- 0.71 to 0.95, and internal consistencies were excellent, ranging from 0.86 to 0.96. This suggests that changing the factor structure might be useful for improving the validity of the instrument in other cultures/languages. However, this improvement would be gained at the expense of comparability between studies on different cultures among each other.

Aside from reflecting truly different constructs between the populations studied, diverging results between this and the other studies can also be due to a systematic measurement error caused by method variance. Method variance is a systematic error attributable to the measurement process including scales, items, response formats, response behaviors and survey settings (Podsakoff et al. 2003).

Divergent validity of part II was slightly higher than in the original version, since only two dimensions were correlated with trait positive or negatives affect. The moderate correlation of $r_s=0.45$ between negative affect and emotional representations was also found by Moss-Morris et al. (2002) (r=0.54), suggesting that a considerable amount of variance in the emotional reaction towards illness is accounted for by trait negative affect. This relationship was expected despite findings about cultural variations in emotions (Mesquita/Frijda 1992) since the affect state dimensions represented by the PANAS are related to traits of positive and negative emotional reactivity (Tellegen 1985) and hence, naturally, are related to the emotional representations dimension of the IPQ-R.

4.3.3 IPQ-R part III

Participants had no difficulties in giving responses to part III of the IPQ-R. Item difficulty was satisfactory since responses given for each item were distributed over the entire scale. However, the respective four-factor structures identified by Moss-Morris et al. (2002) and Kocaman et al. (2007) could not be confirmed. Instead, exploratory factor analysis applying different extraction criteria revealed a three-factor solution. This solution, derived on the basis of statistical and theoretical considerations, produced acceptable results with the three factors discriminating well against each other. Different reasons could be responsible for this diverging finding. First, common method variance as mentioned above could have created differences between the structures that are not due to true conceptual differences in the beliefs of the study participants, but which simply reflect effects from the measurement process applied. Similarly, the small sample size could have underpowered the analysis and, hence, distorted the extraction of factors. Second, the divergent factor structures could reflect true differences between Turkish migrants residing in Germany and Turks residing in Turkey as regards causal attributions (Faltermaier 2001).

Efficiency and reasonableness of the IPQ-R is limited since it has a rather high testtaker burden and provides only slow assessment. However, its test utility is high since they allow an in-depth assessment of very important psychological constructs.

4.3.4 Brief IPQ

The Brief IPQ performed well and gained similar results as the original version. Due to its single-item approach, item scores are easy to interpret, because increases in these scores represent linear increases in the respective beliefs. These properties—easy application and interpretation—make the Brief IPQ a valuable instrument for clinical practice. Convergent and divergent validity of the Brief IPQ were acceptable and correlations between the IPQ-R and the Brief IPQ were identified as expected. Relationships between both instruments were similar to those in the original validation study (Broadbent et al. 2006). However, it has to be noted and considered that the convergent validity was assessed by means of a suboptimal version of the IPQ-R.

Correlations between IPQ-R and Brief IPQ dimensions, in part, were slightly lower than in the original validation study. The relationship between the timeline and control dimensions was not significant. The correlation with the control dimensions was also lowest among all correlations in the original validation study of the Brief IPQ. It is known from research on self-efficacy that a close link exists between the measurement of control beliefs and self-efficacy, especially when a single item approach is used (Maurer/Pierce 1998). However, unlike in the original validation, self-efficacy could not be assessed as a supporting validity measure which is why validity of the control scale can only be assumed, supported by experiences from the original validation.

In general, the same causal attributions as with the IPQ-R were identified by means of the Brief IPQ. This is in line with results from a study by French et al. (2001) who found out that causal attributions as measured by a pre-set scale were almost equal to responses given by individuals to open-ended questions. Furthermore, the current results show the advantage of an open-ended response format over the IPQ-R part III because a significant number of responses given were not covered by the attributions pre-listed in the questionnaire. This corresponds to Broadbent et al's (2006) findings. The way of analyzing the causal attributions in the Brief IPQ depends on the research purpose. In clinical practice, the responses could be directly addressed in personal contact. In research settings, only the top-rated cause could be considered or the responses could be grouped into higher ordered clusters.

Regarding secondary quality criteria of psychometric instruments, the Brief IPQ performs better than the IPQ-R. It is more efficient since it allows a faster assessment, easier application and analysis, and is more reasonable due to its brevity and the reduction of test-taker burden. Despite measuring the same aspects as the IPQ-R, test utility of the Brief IPQ is high, since measurement is quicker and requires fewer resources.

In the Brief IPQ, fewer problems with misunderstanding were encountered by participants as compared to the IPQ-R. This may be attributable to the translation process of the Brief IPQ that considered the characteristics of Turkish migrants.

•

4.3.5 Strengths and limitations of the case study

Strengths

The study outlined in this book is one of the few empirical examples that translated and validated an existing self-report instrument in Turkish migrants residing in Germany and is the first study dealing with the validation of the IPQ-R and the Brief IPQ in this population group. The translation process of the Brief IPQ comprised a forward and backward translation and followed translation guidelines. The adapted and translated instrument was tested in a small sample and revised according to respondents' opinions prior to its implementation in this study. Although the study applied exploratory factor analysis instead of confirmatory factor analysis, sophisticated factor analytic techniques were utilized to test the factor structure of the instrument in question. Interviews were conducted by interviewers proficient in Turkish language and experienced in conducting interviews. With one exception all interviewers had a background in health research and all had both cultural and social experiences in the Turkish community. The response rate in the rehabilitation clinics was quite high, supporting representativity for migrants in this rehabilitation setting.

Limitations

Aside from strengths, several limitations could be identified. While some are due to external factors and difficult to modify, others give valuable advice about changes that need to be implemented prior to a full-scale validation study.

The *settings chosen for recruitment*, self-help groups (SHGs) and rehabilitation clinics, and the way the sample was drawn can be criticized in different respects. First, SHGs and rehabilitation clinics are not representative for chronically ill Turkish migrants residing in Germany. In both settings, different selection processes are involved that undermine representativity. Studies on Turkish migrants have shown that, for them, SHGs, unlike the own family system and network of friends and neighbors, do not play a relevant role as institutions for seeking help outside the medical system (Eckert et al. 2006; Naz 2006). In part, this could be associated with a low number of SHGs offering services tailored to migrants and populations with a low socio-economic status as has frequently been criticized (Kofahl 2007; Bobzien et al. 2002). Consequently, those participating in SHGs may experience barriers less restrictive and hence are different from others not participating (e.g. regarding the degree of integration and the size of social network, etc.). Although, in the current study, patients were recruited from SHGs which offered services for Turkish migrants and which were led by Turkish speaking personnel, it is highly likely that only a selected group of patients participated, because different factors could have influenced access to self-help groups. For example, sessions were attended by females only. Although a few self-help groups exist that target Turkish migrant males, these groups are only poorly attended and no meetings took place during the time of patient recruitment. Aside from sex, other selection criteria could be age, place of residence, and disease state. Attending sessions requires sufficient mobility to get to places where meetings are held. Limited mobility due to poor infrastructure or poor health could prevent some persons from participating. Similarly, attendees and non-attendees could differ regarding their social support. As mentioned above, the utilization of self-help and lay system services among migrants is quite high. However, this rather concerns family and friends than self-help groups. Consequently, it would be possible that those attending SHGs compensate missing social support from the family, friends, or neighbors, and thus differ in a factor highly relevant for coping behavior. As mentioned previously, illness representations are also associated with a number of coping strategies and with the utilization of different health services. Although no studies exist examining the role of illness beliefs for the attendance at self-help groups in migrants, it can be assumed that both attendees and non-attendees hold particular beliefs that distinguish them from each other. This and the previous assumption are supported by studies dealing with similar aspects in different populations. In a Dutch study on 238 prostate cancer patients, Voerman et al. (2007) found out that age, lack of social support, positive attitudes, and high perceived control were associated with the intention to participate in "social support groups" (this terms refers to self-help groups led by laymen or professionals). Perceived control and the severity of disease symptoms were associated with actual participation. Comparable results were obtained by Sherman et al. (2008) who studied 425 male and female patients of different malignancies. They found out that perceived severity of illness and geographic residence where significantly associated with SHG participation, even after adjusting for other variables.

Similar aspects hold true for rehabilitation clinics, where some individuals experience barriers to attendance more impassable than others. Hence, in the present case, Turkish migrants that have been surveyed in these clinics are not representative for all chronically ill Turkish migrants residing in Germany. As could be seen in chapter 3, illness perceptions are related to patients' decision whether or not to participate in rehabilitation programs. Newer studies on different patient populations found out that non-attendance is associated with low income, single living, long travel time, low family support, and less severe symptoms (Nielsen et al. 2008; Higgins et al. 2008; Sabit et al. 2008; Hagan et al. 2007).

Consequently, regarding the selection process it can be concluded that no representativity for all chronically ill individuals with a Turkish migration background could be reached. Therefore, the external validity of the current study is limited, since results are only applicable to Turkish migrant populations of rehabilitation clinics and SHGs that in both cases offer services specifically tailored to Turkish migrants. Additionally, the habit of Turkish migrants to spend their summer in Turkey, may have introduced a slight selection bias, too.

Criteria for inclusion and exclusion of participants were not very strict resulting in a quite diverse sample and minor problems regarding patients' suitability for the participation in the survey. Turkish language instruments adapted for use in Turkish migrants residing in Germany can only be applied to those individuals whose primary language is Turkish. Considering this requirement, the primary language criterion should have been followed more strictly. Besides, the information on language proficiency was not based on self-report, but on information given by the clinic personnel. Additionally, although these local coordinators were instructed to recruit all participants with a Turkish migration background and to inform the principal investigator of patients not eligible for survey due to their health state, it cannot be ruled out that pre-selection during the recruitment process biased the results. Furthermore, not all patients admitted to the clinic during the recruitment period were recruited and surveyed. The survey only included those met in the clinic on the six days on which interviews took place throughout the 2.5-month period. Additionally, unlike other studies applying a version of the IPQ-R, no particular illness groups had been preselected. Instead, all Turkish migrant patients with chronic illness admitted to the rehabilitation clinics or attending the SHGs were recruited, resulting in a rather diverse population as regards underlying diseases. Although other validation studies on the IPQ or its subsequent versions also pooled cases from different illness groups to estimate validity (for example, cf. the original validation studies), they had larger subpopulations and, hence, did not run into trouble regarding underpowering of particular sub-groups as might have be the case in the present study.

With regard to the *questionnaire compilation* used, it can be criticized that the SF-12, one of the two secondary instruments used for validation of the IPQ-R and the Brief IPQ, is not suitable for small sample sizes (Ware et al. 1996). Indeed, Ware et al. (1996) showed that the validity of the composite measures of the SF-12 is lower the smaller the size of the sample is. However, the main purpose of including the SF-

12 in this study was to test whether patients experience any problems with filling in this questionnaire in order to resolve possible issues prior to a full-scale validation. In such a study, the SF-12 would play a central role in examining predictive validity, an aspect that had been ignored for the present case a priori. However, aside from testing the usability of this instrument, it was used as an additional measure for divergent validity. Considering the small sample size, the respective result has to be treated with caution. Another important aspect concerns the questionnaire version. For the reasons described in chapter 4.1.3, version 1 of the SF-12 was used. This, however, has several shortcomings. It constricts the calculation of summary measures to the two composite scores PCS and MCS. The scores of the eight underlying dimensions known from the SF-36, e.g. vitality and physical functioning, cannot be computed. Hence, as additional measures to examine divergent validity of the two primary instruments, in the present case, the two composite scores of the SF-12 had to be calculated, while applying a selection of the eight underlying dimensions would have been more appropriate (cf. Weinman et al. 1996; Giardini et al. 2007). Both the SF-12 and the PANAS have been used for the validation of the two primary instruments without prior validation in Turkish migrants. Although both secondary instruments have been psychometrically tested and considered good for the native population in Turkey, it would be wrong to conclude that they perform well for Turkish migrant populations, too. At this point, this limitation can be hardly avoided, since instruments validated for Turkish migrants in Germany are rare.

Podsakoff et al. (2003) list different potential causes of *common method biases* of which some are less but others potentially more important for the current survey. First of all, different common rater effects should be taken into account. Considering the format of the IPQ-R, respondents may have had the tendency to maintain consistency and rationality in their responses to certain similar items. This phenomenon has been described as the "consistency motif" in behavioral research and in particular may come into play when individuals are asked to provide information about their beliefs and attitudes (ibid; Johns 1994). Additionally, social desirability and acquiescence biases, i.e. the tendency of participants to agree or disagree to items disregarding their content—two aspects that play a particular role in minority populations and contributing to systematic differences (Johnson/Vijver 2003)—may have affected the structure of the instrument. Johnson/Vijver (2003) explain these higher values of social desirability by social exclusion, discrimination, and less political rights migrants may experience in the target country. Also, in the current study, it was noticeable that respondents sometimes tended to give vague responses rather than clearly agreeing or disagreeing with a particular statement. This was especially the case in interviewer-administered questionnaires which could be attributed to a feeling of uncertainty and social desirability. Social desirability also plays an important role for item construction, since the way items are worded can reflect desirable attitudes or behaviors, what is referred to as "item social desirability". Although this was minimized by a careful translation of the Brief IPQ and although the translation of the IPQ-R was very close to its original version, it cannot be ruled out that different population groups (in the present case, patients in England/New Zealand/US, in Turkey, and Turkish migrants residing in Germany) experience different degrees of subjective social expectations. Following the explanation of Johnson/Vijver (2003) about the important role of social desirability in minorities, this aspect has to be considered in the interpretation of the results as well. A potential bias also arises from item ambiguity and complexity. Some patients had difficulties in understanding certain items and/or complained about the similarity of certain items. Hence, it is possible that they answered items randomly or systematically using their own heuristics (Peterson 2000).

The *sample size* of this study was limited in order to meet the philosophy of a pilot study. Although it was sufficiently high to perform EFA according to some studies, other studies point out that results may be distorted by errors and less accuracy if the sample size is too small (Osborne/Costello 2004). This might have also been the case here. Hence, the interpretation of the results must consider this possible limitation due to sample size.

The *imputation methods* applied in this study are not regarded as a limitation per se, since many studies have shown the comparability of results gained by analysis on imputed incomplete as compared to complete data. Instead of imputation, future studies could also apply advanced factor analytic techniques designed to deal with missing data (Song/Belin 2008). However, a high number of missing values as in the present study may reduce external validity and needs to be considered in the interpretation of results as well.

By using two different methods of questionnaire administration valuable experience could be gained with regard to the response behavior of Turkish migrants literature has devoted only little attention to. However, pooling responses from differently administered questionnaires could be problematic, since results produced by each method can be inconsistent (Bowling 2005). This has been shown for surveys on different topics, such as alcohol and tobacco use (Wright et al. 1998) or sexual behavior (Couper/Stinson 1999). The inconsistency is larger the more sensitive the research topic is (Lessler/O'Reilly 1997). Although questions asked in this study were less intimate, it cannot be ruled out that SAQ- and IAQ-respondents differed in their response behavior due to social desirability and fear of reprisal. This could also be due to a bias introduced by the interviewers themselves. Additionally, this possible interviewer-bias might not be consistent over all respondents because data was collected by more than one interviewer. Since sensitivity analysis could not be carried out due to the small sample size, it remains unclear to what extent results differed over the five interviewers involved in the data collection process.

5. Outlook: How to proceed from here

Only few methodical experiences are available regarding the use of quantitative instruments in Turkish migrants residing in Germany. We contributed to filling this gap
by testing the IPQ-R and the Brief IPQ in this population on an exploratory basis. Our
findings allow insights into challenges involved in the application of quantitative instruments to migrants. In particular, they highlight obstacles to the administration of
instruments originally developed or adapted for the respective native (i.e. source)
populations.

Participants experienced various problems with completing the Turkish IPQ-R. Disregarding unequal conditions between this and the Turkish validation study, this indicates differences between Turks residing in Turkey and Turkish migrants residing in
Germany that are relevant for psychometric properties of instruments. Consequently,
instruments validated in the former population do not necessarily perform well in the
latter.

In such situations, a separate validation and re-adaptation for Turkish migrants is
necessary. As outlined previously, this aspect is ignored by many studies, making
their results disputable. Considering this requirement, a re-adaptation of the IPQ-R
for Turkish migrants is needed before it can be applied in research on this population
group. Starting points were identified in this study and recommendations about modi-
fying the IPQ-R accordingly will be made in chapter 5.1. Unlike in the Turkish version
of the IPQ-R, the translation process of the Brief IPQ considered the characteristics
of Turkish migrants in Germany. The better performance of the Brief-IPQ as regards
understanding, clarity, and test-taker burden may to a certain extent be attributable to
this migrant-specific adaptation. A thorough investigation by means of a full-scale
validation (chapter 5.1) needs to explore this assumption further.

This case study shows how important it is to appropriately adapt instruments for the
study population. However, in cross-cultural research which aims to make comparisons between population groups with different culture and/or language, the adaptation of instruments may affect the comparability of cross-cultural assessments negatively. Therefore, in these settings, researchers not only need to ensure that instruments are valid and reliable, they also have to make sure that their properties are
equivalent across the populations under study. We will elaborate on this frequently
neglected aspect in chapter 5.2.

5.1 Towards a full-scale validation of the IPQ-R/Brief IPQ

5.1.1 Setting and recruitment process

As outlined previously, patients in SHGs and rehabilitation clinics are subject to different selection processes. Thus these settings are of limited use as recruitment sites
for studies focusing on chronically ill Turkish migrants in general. Unlike these settings, general medical practices are less susceptible to a selection bias and hence

are more adequate to recruit chronically ill Turkish patients. Two general practices with a large number of Turkish migrants among their regular patients have also been contacted in the planning phase of the current study. However, recruitment would have required larger resources because patients would have to be surveyed on a regular basis throughout a long period of time instead of being surveyed in groups on single days as was the case in SHGs and rehabilitation clinics. Also, doctors were concerned about their practice work flow being disturbed by interviewers and did not agree to participate. For this reason, a future validation study first must invest resources to make this setting accessible. Alternatively, patients could be surveyed in hospitals after being admitted for certain events related to their chronic diseases. In this case, the survey procedure could be similar to the situation in the current study, where a clinic-based (or SHG-based) approach was used. Advantages of general hospitals over rehabilitation clinics and SHGs are that they are less prone to selection mechanisms based on patient beliefs and preferences.

Unlike in this study, the type of questionnaire administration should be consistent over all patients. Although the IPQ-R and the Brief IPQ have originally been developed to be self-administered, experiences gained in this study show that this type of administration is inadequate for most Turkish migrants. Instead, a standardized interviewer-administered approach should be used. This was also the case in the Turkish validation by Kocaman et al. (2007). If this approach is chosen, it must be assured that interviews are conducted by trained personnel to preserve instrument objectivity. Consequently, time needed for the training of interviewers should be considered in the planning of the study. Additionally, instructions about the interview procedure should be put down in the study protocol. Special attention should be paid to instructions about anonymity. Other inclusion and exclusion criteria should be equal to this case study.

Factors affecting the motivation of individuals to participate in research are quite complex (Groves et al. 1992). In the current study, motivation was rather low which was also due to the questionnaire length. Aside from improvements of the questionnaire (see below), incentives should be implemented into the recruitment process to enhance motivation. Different studies have shown that the provision of incentives to patients increases the response rate significantly (for instance, cf. the meta-analysis by Edwards et al. 2002 on the role of incentives in postal questionnaires). Incentives could be money, vouchers, a special kind of counseling service, or similar forms of compensation.

5.1.2 Modification of the questionnaire compilation

The questionnaire compilation used in this study has several shortcomings. While some of these can be altered in a future validation study, others are immanent to the research question and can not be addressed. One of the most serious problems is the length of the questionnaire that, in total, consists of 116 items. Although many of these are item batteries using the same response format (e.g. 57 items use 5-point response scales ranging from "I don't think so at all" to "I absolutely think so") test-taker burden with regard to time is comparably high. The time patients needed to complete questionnaires varied considerably. While some patients who filled in questionnaires on their own needed about 20 minutes for completion, others needed twice as long. On average, completion took longer for interviewer-administered questionnaires. However, all of the items currently included in the questionnaire are needed for a proper validation. Hence, it is not possible to create a questionnaire that is more concise. As compared to other validation studies of the IPQ-R that use the SF-36 instead of the SF-12, the current questionnaire compilation can even be considered parsimonious. Whereas a reduction of the total number of items would be unwise, it is nonetheless possible to reduce test-taker burden by improving patient instructions and refining item wordings. Some recommendations will be made in the following.

Disregarding the purpose of this study to serve as a preliminary step towards a full-scale validation, any studies aiming to validate (psychometric) instruments for migrant populations have to face the shortcoming that secondary instruments required for validation—such as the SF-12 and the PANAS in the present case—themselves are often not appropriately tested in migrant populations. This limitation is hardly avoidable and therefore needs to be addressed in the interpretation of the results, especially because findings indicating validity problems in the primary instrument could in fact be the consequence of an inadequate adaptation of the secondary instruments.

SF-12 version 2

For reasons outlined in chapter 4.1.3, the SF-12 version 1, was used as a measure of health-related quality of life. However, version 1 has many shortcomings with regard to its interpretability. It was professionally adapted for Turkish culture and language and formally validated in the Turkish population of Turkey. However, due to a high-standard language style and complicated wordings, test-taker burden for this questionnaire was, nonetheless, high and comprehensibility in Turkish migrants limited. For some time, an official adaptation of the SF-12 version 2 is available over QualityMetric Inc. (2008). Although it has not been formally validated in a Turkish population, it holds some essentials improvements over version 1. Not only does it allow an adequate representation of the eight health-related quality of life dimensions of the SF-36, but it has also undergone a methodical refinement and its language style is much plainer and more basic as compared to version 1. This makes it more suitable for the application in Turkish migrants residing in Germany which is also the reason why version 2 should be given preference over version 1 for a future full-scale validation study.

IPQ-R

Similarly, considering patients' feedback and the experiences gained by the research team, some modifications should be applied to the translation of the IPQ-R. While the entire translation of the IPQ-R into Turkish (see http://www.uib.no/ipq/) can be regarded as very proper and accurately representing the original version, at some points it also uses a language style that is difficult to understand for individuals with little formal education in Turkish language and little exposition to modern Turkish language usage. Although the version provided by Kocaman et al. (2007) has been tested and validated, applying some easy tweaking and finishing touches would allow a better understanding of the questionnaire by Turkish migrant patients and enhance comprehensibility without compromising the structure set by the original version.

Despite being worded very clearly using everyday vocabulary, the dual structure of the *IPQ-R part I* did not become clear to participants. Replacing *olup olmadığı* by *görüp görmediğiniz* to stress that patients are asked about their own opinion could enhance patients' understanding. Also, *mide şikayetleri* should be given preference over *mide yakınmaları* (both referring to stomach troubles) because unlike the first, the latter is a less common Turkish noun. Similarly, *uyku bozukluğu* is a better representation of "disturbed sleep" or "sleep disorder" than *uyku güçlükleri* and thus should be preferred. Moreover, additional measures to the layout could be applied to enhance patients' understanding. In any case, further pre-testing is necessary.

Some improvement can also be applied to the *IPQ-R part II*. By means of little modifications, items can be adjusted to the plainer language style of migrants without compromising the comparability to the original version. These changes include the replacement of high-standard words by everyday terms (i.e. *muhtemelen* by *galiba* in item C2, both meaning "probably"; *sonuçları var* by *yükü oluyor* in item C10, both referring to financial burden, *seyri* by *gidişi* both referring to the course of illness). Confusion also existed over the similarity of certain items. This was especially true for items C34 and C35. While in the English version individuals are asked to indicate the degree of their consent to the statements *"I get depressed when I think about my illness"* (C34) and *"When I think about my illness I get upset"* (C35), respectively, the Turkish version uses the adjectives *çökkün* and *üzgün* that many migrants regard as synonymous in Turkish language. In high-standard Turkish, the latter means rather "sad" than "upset". To avoid confusion, the adjective *sinirli* ("upset, nervous") could be used, although it is has to be noted that an adequate adaptation is difficult, since subtle nuances between the two words in English language cannot be properly represented in Turkish language.

As mentioned previously, Turkish language applies agglutination to form words. Due to this grammatical characteristic, the lowest (*"Kesinlikle böyle düşünmüyorum"*, i.e. "I don't think so at all") and highest (*"Kesinlikle böyle düşünüyorum"*, i.e. "I absolutely think so") as well as the second lowest (*"Böyle düşünmüyorum"*, i.e. "I don't think so") and second highest (*"Böyle düşünüyorum"*, i.e. "I think so") labels of the response continuum for part II and III differ only by means of the negation particle *mü* (or *mi*, *mı*, or *mu* depending on vowel harmony) which is an infix between verb stem and pronoun. Consequently, positive and negative statements can easily be confused as occasionally happened during the survey. It cannot be ruled out that other cases of misunderstanding remained unnoticed by the research team. This problem is never addressed in other questionnaires. For example, the Turkish version of the Short Social Support Questionnaire (*Kurzform des Fragebogens zur sozialen Unterstützung, F-SozU K-14;* Fydrich et al. 2007) uses *"kesinlikle uymuyor – pek uymuyor – kısmen uymuyor – uyuyor – kesinlikle uyuyor"* as labels for response categories bearing the same potential for misunderstanding. While special highlighting could be applied as a layout measure to reduce the likelihood of a mix-up, the only possibility to prevent confusion would be the use of different labels that consist of auxiliary rather than full verbs. An example is implemented in the Turkish adaptation of the General Perceived Self-Efficacy Scale *(Skala zur Allgemeinen Selbstwirksamkeitserwartung, SWE)* by Yeşilay et al. (no date). The author uses the labels *"doğru değil – biraz doğru – daha doğru – tümüyle doğru" ("not true – somewhat true – more true – absolutely true")* following the original response categories that are labeled *"Not true at all – Hardly true – Moderately true – Exactly true"* in the English version (Schwarzer/Jerusalem 1995). Labels for the first and second part of the IPQ-R could be similar, e.g. *"Kesinlikle doğru değil – Doğru değil – Kararsızım – Doğru – Tümüyle doğru" ("Not true at all – Not true – In am not sure – True – Absolutely true")*. Although these labels do not accurately represent the original questionnaire format, they could be implemented in light of the misunderstandings that occasionally occurred with the more accurate full verb solution. As addressed previously, most probably as a result of the grammatical phenomenon outlined above, patients did not notice that item C36 was reversed as could be concluded from its negative factor loading and negative item-total correlation. This could be easily prevented in future studies by highlighting the negation particle of this item.

As regards *part III*, the noun *kalıtsal* referring to "heredity" can be replaced or complemented by the straight forward term *genetik* that is better known by patients.

Brief IPQ

Fewer stumbling blocks were identified in the translation of the Brief IPQ which could be explained by the consideration of migrant-specific characteristics in the translation process. As mentioned in chapter 2, an alternative translation of the Brief IPQ was available on the internet after this study had been completed. This alternative translation slightly differs from the current translation. While it can be considered better in terms of language quality for some items, other wordings are problematic. With regard to the introduction part, the short pre-test implemented in the present translation process showed that respondents needed additional information on how to respond on the 11-point linear scale. For some individuals it was not clear that the scale has to be interpreted as an intensity rating from low to high. Consequentially, the introduction of the questionnaire should be complemented by an additional explanation. This study showed that by means of this addition, participants had considerably fewer problems in answering questions.

Question 1, 2, and 3 are almost identical between the present and the version by Olfaz. In the third question, Olfaz used the verb *hissetmek (to feel)*. For the reasons outlined in chapter 4.1.1, in the present version *düşünmek (to think)* has been given preference over *hissetmek* because it is more consistent with the original version, less susceptible to misunderstandings, and is also used in other questions of the translated Brief IPQ. The seventh question of the alternative version does not adequately represent the original English version. It is *"Hastalığınızın ne olduğunu ne kadar iyi anladınız?"* which means *"How well did you understand what your illness is?"* while the original version reads *"How well do you feel you understand your illness?"* which is more properly represented by the translation in the present version asking *"Hastalığınızı ne kadar iyi anladığınızı düşünüyorsunuz?"*. Olfaz translated the fourth item by *"Tedavinizin hastalığınıza ne ölçüde yardımcı olabileceğini düşünüyor-*

sunuz?" and the sixth by *"Hastalığınız için ne kadar endişelisiniz?"* which is very similar to and equally as good as the current translation. The last item has been translated as *"Hastalığınız duygusal olarak sizi ne kadar etkilemekte? (ör: Sizi sinirli, ürkek, üzüntülü veya çökkün yapıyor mu?)"* which is also very similar to the translation in the current study. The choice of the word *çökkün* is perhaps nearer to everyday language and could be used instead of the synonymous *depresif*. The abbreviation *ör* (equivalent to English *e.g.*) for *örneğin (for example)* is problematic because it might be unknown to participants not proficient in Turkish-language reading and writing. Olfaz' translation of the fifth question *("Hastalığınıza bağlı şikayetleri hangi ölçüde yaşıyorsunuz?")* is slightly better than the current one, because it reflects the original version better and has been translated more idiomatically. However, the word *şikayet (complaint, grouch, grouse)* should be replaced by *belirti (symptom)* as the original asks for the latter. Differences between the current and the alternative Turkish translation also exist as regards the endpoint labels. In the alternative version, endpoint labels have been translated directly and kept as short as they are in the original English version. However, by forming complete sentences as in this study understanding can be easily enhanced without violating the structure of the original version. The usage of the adjective *ömür boyu (lifelong, all/throughout one's life)* in the endpoint label of question 2 as suggested by Olfaz should be given preference over the adjective *her zaman (always, all along)* chosen in the current translation, since it is closer to the original. Similarly, the alternative endpoints *"Tedavim hiç yardımcı değil – Tedavim oldukça yardımcı"* and *"Duygusal olarak hiç etkilemiyor – Duygusal olarak çok etkiliyor"* could be used in questions 4 and 8, respectively. Labels for question 5 have to be adjusted accordingly (*"Hiçbir belirtilerim olmuyor – Çok ciddi belirtilerim oluyor"*) if the alternative translation is to be used. By implementing the modifications outlined above, the usability of the current translation of the Brief IPQ can be further improved.

5.1.3 Study design

The study design of a full-scale validation would base on the design applied in the current study, but, in addition, would include a prospective component to assess test-retest reliability and predictive validity. Also, to apply a confirmatory analysis framework in order to assess structural validity, at least 300 to 350 patients should be recruited for the study. Following other IPQ-R validation studies, it is possible to recruit patients from more than one disease group, i.e. cardiovascular diseases (including an MI sub-sample), diabetes, and cancer. Combining CFA with a single-disease approach as was done by Hagger/Orbell (2005) for the CFA validation of the IPQ-R in a cervical screening context would be desirable, however, would require a much longer recruitment period.

After the conduction of a cross-sectional baseline survey similar to the one carried out in the present case, a sub-sample of 80 patients would be followed-up and re-surveyed after six months in order to assess stability of the IPQ-R and the Brief IPQ over time. This test-retest reliability would be measured by correlating the IPQ-R/Brief IPQ scores obtained at the two time points (baseline vs. six months later). Another sub-sample of 80 MI patients would be followed-up for a three-month period in order to test predictability of certain key outcomes following MI, e.g. quality of life as measured by the SF-12 (see Fig. 11). Since sub-groups would be large enough, also known-group validity could be assessed. Furthermore, the secondary test quality criterion of fairness should be paid more attention to (Kubinger 2005). Optionally, in the two sub-groups, baseline validity measures could also be assessed longitudinally (Liang 2000; see Holtby/Razmjou 2005 for an example of a study assessing cross-sectional and longitudinal validity of an instrument).

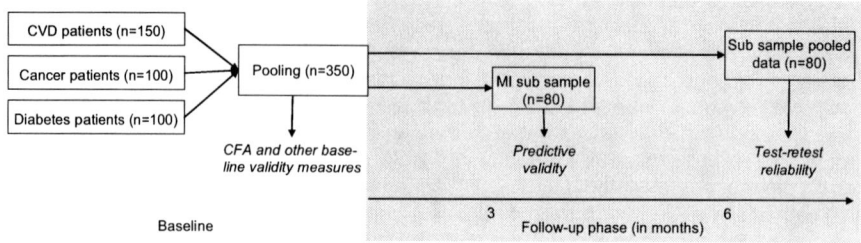

Fig. 11: Recommended design of a full-scale validation study (Source: Own data)

5.2 Ensuring comparability in research across cultures

Researchers working on cross-cultural research topics not only need to rely on instruments that are able to measure variables of interest with high validity and reliability within one population, they also have to make sure that measurements taken with these instruments are comparable across different cultural groups. In this respect, the degree to which an instrument is adapted for a particular population may interfere with the degree of cross-cultural comparability.

In a review article, Herdman et al. (1997) identified four different approaches to cross-cultural adaptation: The *relativist approach* maintains that it is impossible to use standardized instruments across cultures. The *naïve approach* translates instruments by means of a simple one-way translation process. Similar to the naïve approach, the *absolutist approach* maintains that culture has very little impact on the construct measured—a quite questionable assumption, as outlined in this book. This approach focuses on translation only, but applies more sophisticated translation techniques comprising one or several forward- and back-translation cycles. Finally, the *universalist* approach does not assume that constructs are stable across cultures. Instead, it calls for examining whether constructs which particular instruments are supposed to assess are the same in all populations under study and whether the instruments in question provide comparable results across these populations.

5.2.1 The role of linguistic equivalence

All instruments applied in this study were developed in the US, New Zealand, or Western Europe. Since every society develops a particular language code, concepts, words, and descriptions are not necessarily comparable between different cultures (Hoffmeyer-Zlotnik 1985). Hence, possible incompatibilities arising from the 'Western' origin of these instruments and their underlying frameworks are relevant. In some aspects they may be unknown to non-Western societies unless culturally adapted, thus affecting linguistic equivalence of the translated as compared to the original version of the questionnaires.

Linguistic equivalence tells whether the original and the translated words and items have the same meaning. According to Schöneberg (1985), linguistic equivalence is influenced by the lexical correspondence of original and translated words, the cultural specificity and the frequency of the usage of expressions in the original and the target language, as well as the syntactical context in which expressions and words are applied.

The problem of poor linguistic equivalence is well known and especially becomes relevant when idioms are used. It has to be faced in the translations of different instruments that apply such expression in their original versions. The item *"Have you felt downhearted and blue?"* from the SF-36, for example, is hard to translate into other languages due to the special meaning of the term "blue". As another example, the Beliefs About Medicine Questionnaire (Horne et al. 1999) asks respondents to rate the statement *"All medicines are poison"*. Research has shown that this notion does not emerge as a relevant representation in languages other than English (cf. Horne 1997, Fallsberg 1991), simultaneously making the usage of this item in other language questionable and challenging its cross-cultural comparability in case this item is deleted.

Similar problems arise in the IPQ-R. While the item *"My illness is a mystery to me"* has been translated into Italian (Giardini et al. 2007) and Spanish (Vázquez et al. 2007), literally (*"La mia malattia è un mistero per me"* and *"Mi hipertensión es un misterio para mi"*, respectively), Kocaman et al. (2007) translated the item as *"Hastalığım bana anlamsız geliyor"* (*"My illness is meaningless to me"*) into Turkish indicating that no equivalent translation exists in the Turkish language. These kinds of divergences between instruments and their translations are difficult to avoid and immanent to the topic of cultural adaptation, because they reflect the differences in cultures and languages. They are the larger the more the culture and language of origin differs from the culture and language of the target adaptation. In the present case—an instrument developed in Western societies in English language and adapted for Turkish-language migrants—there are considerable differences in both culture as well as language family (Indo-Germanic vs. Turkic). Despite these differences, Kocaman et al. (2007) used a rather literal translation for the IPQ-R. This is good regarding comparability if its properties before and after the translation remain equal, but critical if the translated instrument does not represent the underlying framework as well as the original version. According to the Turkish validation study, it does in chronically ill Turks in Turkey. As has been pointed out in chapter 2, it is known that Turkish migrants residing in Germany and the native Turkish population of Turkey differ with regard to socio-demographic factors and may also be different regarding their cultural belief system which depends on the degree of secularization and modernization. Also, various challenges for research emerge from changes to language usage through the process of migration (Mangalam 1968; Kerswill 1994). As for the situation in Germany, these challenges for example are reflected in the heterogeneity of language usage among Turkish migrants. While first-generation migrants often have little or no competency in German, this changes in subsequent generations who grow up in Germany (Esser 2006). As is well known from national and international migration research (e.g. Alba et al. 2002), this often results in a language shift through which, with increasing duration of stay and subsequent generations, competency of German exceeds competency in Turkish (Esser 2006). Counterintuitive findings of the study presented here as compared to the Turkish validation might in part be attributable to this phenomenon.

5.2.2 Beyond linguistic equivalence

By focusing on wording in the first place, recommendations made in this study mainly concentrated on the role of possible language differences between the two populations leading to difference in psychometric properties. However, other dimensions of cross-cultural comparability are relevant as well and need to be considered by researchers applying a universalist approach.

Herdman et al. (1998) identified the following properties an instrument must offer to a certain degree before it can be applied in cross-cultural research. Apart from linguistic equivalence (also called *semantic equivalence*) these are:

- *Conceptual equivalence* (also called *external construct equivalence*). It tells whether an instrument, in each culture/population group under study, has the same relationship to the construct it is supposed to measure and whether this construct is conceptualized equally well in all study groups.

- *Operational equivalence,* means that the same type of questionnaire administration, text format etc. can be used across different populations.

- *Measurement equivalence* (also called *internal construct equivalence*) can be assumed when different versions of an instrument show the same psychometric properties.

- *Item equivalence* can, on the one hand, be considered a part of conceptual equivalence in the way that it concerns equal meanings of items across cultures; on the other hand, it is a component of measurement equivalence referring to the equal relationship of items and scales across different populations (cf. also Berry et al. 1992).

As illustrated in Fig. 12, conceptual, linguistic, operational, item and measurement equivalence together form the *functional equivalence* of an instrument. It can be defined as "the extent to which an instrument does what it is supposed to do equally well in two or more cultures" (Herdman et al. 1998, p. 331). Different guidelines for cross-cultural adaptation exist assisting researchers in constructing functionally equivalent instruments (e.g. Peters/Passchier 2006; Beaton et al. 2000; Guillemin et al. 1993).

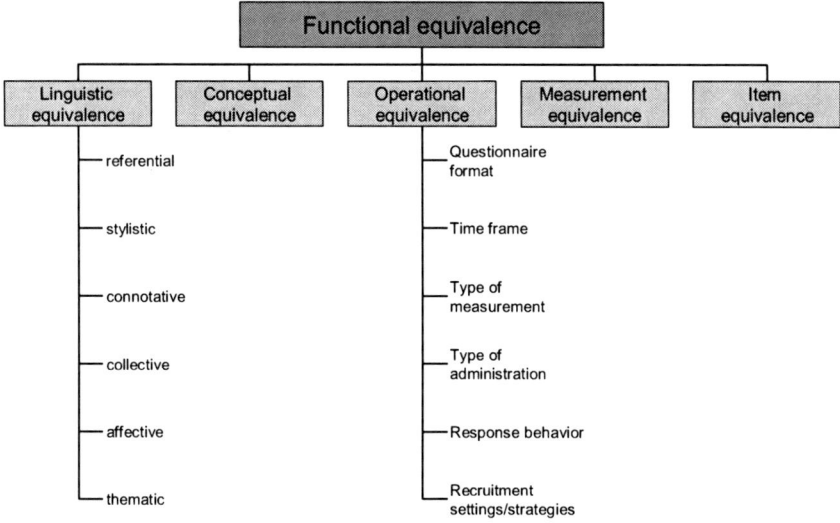

Fig. 12: The components of functional equivalence of an instrument (Own illustration based on Herdman et al. 1998)

Prior to the application of instruments in cross-cultural research projects, researchers need to make sure that these instruments are functionally equivalent across the populations they study. They need to examine whether instruments represent constructs equally well and whether theoretical models representing these constructs are transferable across their study groups. For operational equivalence, researchers need to assess whether the same survey methods regarding format, time frame, measurement as well as mode and setting of administration can be applied across the populations studied and whether these populations differ in response behavior. Furthermore, the feasibility of the recruitment in particular settings and by means of particular strategies across cultures needs to be examined. If the analysis shows that for each population under study different methods for operationalization must be applied, possible consequences of these differences must be described and considered in the analysis. Finally, researchers need to examine the measurement equivalence of instruments. Apart from testing and comparing the criterion and content validity, this comprises comparing the factorial validity and internal consistency of instruments as well as testing the hypotheses that for all groups under study the same factor pattern can be extracted, that corresponding factor loadings are equal and that their latent traits can be measured with the same accuracy.

Only by carefully assessing functional equivalence, researchers can disclose possible differences in the psychometric properties of their instruments which may limit the comparability between their study populations and distort their findings. Current literature considers the examination of functional equivalence especially important when it comes to the adaptation of instruments to different languages and cultures. The results of our case study suggest that it may also be a relevant aspect in migrant health research when researchers use the translated and validated instrument versions of the respective native (i.e. source) populations. Since possible biases arising from functionally inequivalent instruments usually are not taken into account, findings generated that way must be treated with caution.

Which dimensions of functional equivalence may be affected by this transfer of same language instruments in particular, is subject of our ongoing research. Results will allow to illustrate limitations as well as challenges of this practice. In addition, the findings will provide a sound basis for thorough recommendations concerning the adequate application of quantitative instruments in migrant health research.

References

Adler, Y., Rauchfleisch, U., Müllejans, R. (1996): Die Bedeutung der Konzepte zu Krankheitsursachen und Behandlungserwartungen in der ersten Behandlungsphase. Psychotherapie, Psychosomatik, Medizinische Psychologie 46, 321-326.

Akarçay, M., Kizilay, A., Miman, M. C., Cokkeser, Y., Ozturan, O. (2003): Endoskopik sinüs cerrahisinin yaşam kalitesi üzerine etkisi [The effect of endoscopic sinus surgery on quality of life]. Kulak Burun Bogaz Ihtis Degisi 11, 65-71.

Akbiyik, I.D., Berksun, O. E., Sumbuloglu, V., Sentürk, V., Priebe, S. (2008): Quality of life of Turkish patients with depression in Ankara and in Berlin. European Psychiatry Suppl 1, 4-9.

Alba, R.D., Logan, J. R., Lutz, A., Stults, B. (2002): Only English by the third generation? Loss and preservation of the mother tongue among the grandchildren of contemporary immigrants. Demography 39, 467-484.

Allender, S., Scarborough, P., Peto, V., Ryner, M., Leal, J., Luengo-Fernandez, R., Gray, A. (2008): European cardiovascular disease statistics. 2008 edition. Brussels: European Heart Network. [Online] URL: http://www.ehnheart.org/files/statistics%202008%20web-161229A.pdf (Accessed: Apr. 01,2010)

Amann, G., Wipplinger, R. (1998): Die Relevanz subjektiver Krankheitstheorien in der Gesundheitsförderung. In: Amann, G., Wipplinger, R. (Eds.): Gesundheitsförderung: Ein multidimensionales Tätigkeitsfeld. Tübingen: Dgvt-Verlag, 153-175.

American Psychological Association (2003): Guidelines on multicultural education, training, research practice, and organizational change for psychologists. American Psychologist 58, 377-402.

Anagnostopoulos, F., Spanea, E. (2005): Assessing illness representations of breast cancer. A comparison of patients with healthy and benign controls. Journal of Psychosomatic Research 58, 327-334.

Anastasi, A. (1972): Psychological testing. London: Collier-Macmillan.

Ano, G.G., Vasconcelles, E. B. (2005): Religious coping and psychological adjustment to stress: a meta-analysis. Journal of Clinical Psychology 61, 461-480.

Arthur, S., Nazroo, S. (2003): Designing fieldwork strategies and materials. In: Ritchie, J., Lewis, J. (Eds.): Qualitative Research Practice. London: Sage, 109-137.

Aydin, H., Halm, D., Sen, F. (2003): "Euro-Islam". Das neue Islamverständnis der Muslime in der Migration. Essen: Stiftung Zentrum für Türkeistudien.

Backus, A. (2006): Turkish as an immigrant language in Europe. In: Bhatia, T.K., Ritchie, W.C. (Eds.): The handbook of bilingualism. Balden: Blackwell, 689-724.

Baggaley, R.F., Ganaba, R., Filippi, V., Kere, M., Marshall, T., Sombie, I., Storeng, K. T., Patel, V. (2007): Detecting depression after pregnancy: the validity of the K10 and K6 in Burkina Faso. Tropical Medicine and International Health 12, 1225-1229.

Bandura, A. (1977): Social learning theory. Englewood Cliffs: Prentica-Hall.

Barnes, L., Moss-Morris, R., Kaufusi, M. (2004): Illness beliefs and adherence in diabetes mellitus: a comparison between Tongan and European patients. New Zealand Medical Journal 117, U743.

Bartlett, C., Davey, P., Dieppe, P., Doyal, L., Ebrahim, S., Egger, M. (2003): Women, older persons, and ethnic minorities: factors associated with their inclusion in randomised trials of statins 1990 to 2001. Heart 89, 327-328.

Beaton, D.E., Bombardier, C., Guillemin, F., Ferraz, M. B. (2000): Guidelines for the process of cross-cultural adaptation of self-report measures. Spine 25, 3186-3191.

Becker, H. (1984): Die Bedeutung der subjektiven Krankheitstheorie des Patienten für die Arzt-Patienten-Beziehung. Psychotherapie, Psychosomatik, medizinische Psychologie 34, 313-321.

Benyamini, Y., Gozlan, M., Kokia, E. (2008): Women's and men's perceptions of infertility and their associations with psychological adjustment: A dyadic approach. British Journal of Health Psychology.

Berg, G. (2001): Subjektive Krankheitskonzepte - eine kommunikative Voraussetzung für die Arzt-Patientin-Interaktion. In: David, M., Borde, T., Kentenich, H. (Eds.): Migration und Gesundheit: Zustandsbeschreibung und Zukunftsmodelle. Frakfurt am Main: Mabuse, 81-94.

Bernstein, B. (1971): Class, Codes and Control. London: Paladin.

Berry, J.W., Poortinga, Y.H., Segall, M.H., Dasen, P.R. (1992): Cross-cultural psychology: Research and application. Cambridge: Cambridge University Press.

Bobzien, M., Hönigschmid, C., Stark, W. (2002): Entwicklungen und Trends in der gesundheitsbezogenen Selbsthilfe. Handlungsempfehlungen für die Zukunft der Selbsthilfe. Essen/München: Private publishing house.

Boey, K.W. (1999): Cross-validation of a short form of the CES-D in Chinese elderly. International Journal of Geriatric Psychiatry 14, 608-617.

Boos-Nünning, U. (1986): Lebenssituation und Deutungsmuster türkischer Mädchen in der Bundesrepublik Deutschland. In: Yakut, A., Reich, H.H., Neumann, U., Boos-Nünning, U. (Eds.): Zwischen Elternhaus und Arbeitsamt: Türkische Jugendliche suchen einen Beruf. Berlin: 67-106.

Boswell, C. (2005): Migration in Europe. A paper prepared for the Policy Analysis and Research Programme of the Global Commission on International Migration. Geneva: Global Commission on International Migration.

Bowling, A. (2005): Mode of questionnaire administration can have serious effects on data quality. Journal of Public Health 27, 281-291.

Brace, I., Adams, K. (2006): An introduction to market & social Research: Planning & using research tools & techniques. London: Kogan Page.

Brewer, N.T., Chapman, C. B., Brownlee, S., Leventhal, E. A. (2002): Cholesterol control, medication adherence and illness cognition. Journal of Health Psychology 7, 433-447.

Broadbent, E., Petrie, K. J., Main, J., Weinman, J. (2006): The brief illness perception questionnaire. Journal of Psychosomatic Research 60, 631-637.

Brucks, U., Wahl, W. B. (2003): Unter-, Über-, Fehlversorgung? Bedarfslücken und Strukturprobleme in der ambulanten Gesundheitsversorgung für Migrantinnen und Migranten. In: Borde, T., David, M. (Eds.): Gut versorgt? Migrantinnen und Migranten im Gesundheits- und Sozialwesen. Frankfurt/Main: Mabuse, 15-33.

Bryant, F. B. (2000): Assessing the validity of measurement. In: Grimm, L.G., Yarnold, P.R. (Eds.): Reading and understanding MORE multivariate statistics. Washington: American Psychological Association, 99-146.

Bryjak, G. J., Soroka, M. P. (1997): Sociology cultural diversity in a changing world. Boston: Allyn and Bacon.

Brzoska, P., Razum, O. (2009): Krankheitsbewältigung bei Menschen mit Migrationshintergrund im Kontext von Kultur und Religion. Zeitschrift für Medizinische Psychologie 18, 151-161.

Buick, D. L. (1997): Illness representations and breast cancer: Coping with radiation and chemotherapy. In: Petrie, K.J., Weinman, J. (Eds.): Perceptions of health and illness. Current research and applications. Amsterdam: Harwood Academic Publishers, 155-188.

Bulut, S. (2006): Untersuchung zur wohnräumlichen Konzentration von türkischen Migranten in ausgewählten Städten des Ruhrgebietes. Universität Duisburg-Essen, Dissertation.

Bühner, M. (2006): Einführung in die Test- und Fragebogenkonstruktion. München: Pearson Studium.

Byrne, M., Walsh, J., Murphy, A. W. (2005): Secondary prevention of coronary heart disease: patient beliefs and health-related behaviour. Journal of Psychosomatic Research 58, 403-415.

Catell, R.B. (1966): The scree test for number of factors. Multivariate Behavioral Research 1, 246-276.

Chia, L.R., Schlenk, E. A., Dunbar-Jacob, J. (2006): Effect of personal and cultural beliefs on medication adherence in the elderly. Drugs and Aging 23, 191-202.

Christensen, A. J. (2004): Patient adherence to medical treatment regimens. Bridging the gap between behavioral science and biomedicine. New Haven/London: Yale University Press.

Claassen, D., Ascoli, M., Berhe, T., Priebe, S. (2005): Research on mental disorders and their care in immigrant populations: a review of publications from Germany, Italy and the UK. European Psychiatry 20, 540-549.

Clements, F. E. (1932): Primitive concepts of disease. Berkely: University of California Press.

Cochrane Collaboration (2003): Review Manager (RevMan). Version 4.2 for Windows. Copenhagen: The Nordic Cochrane Centre, The Cochrane Collaboration.

Cohen, R. (1978): Ethnicity: Problem and focus in anthropology. Annual Review of Anthropology 7, 379-403.

Cooper, A., Lloyd, G., Weinman, J., Jackson, G. (1999): Why patients do not attend cardiac rehabilitation: role of intentions and illness beliefs. Heart 82, 234-236.

Cooper, A. (2004): Cardiac rehabilitation and recovery from myocardial infarction: The role of patients' illness and treatment beliefs. PhD thesis. University of Brighton.

Corbin, J. M., Strauss, A. L. (1988): Unending work and care. Managing chronic illness at home. San Francisco: Jossey-Bass.

Couper, M.P., Rowe, B. (1996): Evaluation of a computer-assisted self-interview component in a computer-assisted personal interview survey. Public Opinion Quarterly 60, 89-107.

Couper, M.P., Stinson, L. L. (1999): Completion of self-administered questionnaires in a sex survey. The Journal of Sex Research 36, 321-330.

de Vries, H., Brug, J. (1999): Computer-tailored interventions motivating people to adopt health promoting bahaviours: Introduction to a new approach. Patient Education and Counselling 36, 99-105.

Diabetiker Solidaritäts Union (2008): Diabetes-Screening bei Migranten. Diabetiker Solidaritäts Union führt über 2000 Messungen durch. [Online] URL: http://www.diabetesstiftung.de/fileadmin/dds_user/dokumente/DDS_Report_2 00803.pdf (Accessed: Apr. 01,2010)

Dias, S.F., Severo, M., Barros, H. (2008): Determinants of health care utilization by immigrants in Portugal. BMC Health Services Research 8, 207.

Diefenbach, M.A., Leventhal, H. (1996): The common-sense model of illness representation: Theoretical and practical considerations. Journal of Social Distress and the Homeless 5, 11-38.

Dijkstra, A., de Vries, H. (1999): The development of computer-generated tailored interventions. Patient Education and Counselling 36, 193-203.

Duschek, K. J., Weinman, J., Böhm, K., Laue, E., Brückner, G. (2006): Leben in Deutschland - Haushalte, Familien und Gesundheit - Ergebnisse des Mikrozensus 2005. Wiesbaden: Statistisches Bundesamt.

Eberding, A., von Schlippe, A. (2000): Ciğerim yanıyor -- Meine Leber brennt. Systhema 14, 282-292.

Eckert, J., Rommel, A., Weilandt, C. (2006): Gesundheitliche Lage und Gesundheits-verhalten in der Migration. Ergebnisse des Gesundheitsmonitorings der schweizerischen Migrationsbevölkerung 2004. In: Bundsamt für Gesundheit (Ed.): Forschung Migration und Gesundheit im Rahmen der Bundesstrategie "Migration und Gesundheit 2002-2007". Bern: BAG

Edwards, P., Roberts, I., Clarke, M., DiGuiseppi, C., Pratap, S., Wentz, R., Kwan, I. (2002): Increasing response rates to postal questionnaires: systematic review. British Medical Journal 324, 1183.

Emblen, J.D. (1992): Religion and spirituality defined according to current use in nursing literature. Journal of Professional Nursing 8, 41-47.

Ensink, B.J., van Otterloo, D. (1989): A validation study of the DES in the Nether-lands. Dissociation 2, 221-223.

Ercikan, K. (2002): Disentangling sources of differential functioning in multilanguage assessment. International Journal of Testing 2, 199-215.

Esser, H. (2006): Migration, Sprache und Intergration. Berlin: Arbeitsstelle interkultu-relle Konflikte und gesellschaftliche Integration (AKI) und Wissenschaftszent-rum Berlin für Sozialforschung (WZB).

Fallsberg, M. (1991): Reflections on medicines and medication: a qualitative analysis among people on long-term drug regimens. PhD Thesis, Linköping University.

Faltermaier, T., Kühnlein, I., Burda-Viering, M. (1998): Gesundheit im Alltag. Laien-kompetenz in Gesundheitshandeln und Gesundheitsförderung. Weinheim: Ju-venta.

Faltermaier, T., Kühnlein, I. (2000): Subjektive Gesundheitskonzepte im Kontext: Dy-namische Konstruktionen von Gesundheit in einer qualitativen Untersuchung von Berufstätigen. Zeitschrift für Gesundheitspsychologie 8, 137-154.

Faltermaier, T. (2001): Migration und Gesundheit. Fragen und Konzepte aus einer salutogenetischen und gesundheitspsychologischen Perspektive. In: Mar-schalck, P., Wiedl, K.H. (Eds.): Migration und Krankheit. Osnabrück: Rasch, 93-112.

Faltermaier, T. (2002): Gesundheitsvorstellungen und Laienkompetenz. Die Bedeu-tung des Subjektes für die Gesundheitspraxis. Psychomed 14, 149-154.

Faltermaier, T. (2005): Gesundheitspsychologie. Stuttgart.: Kohlhammer.

Figueras, M.J., Weinman, J. (2003): Do similar patient and spouse perceptions of myocardial infarction predict recovery? Psychology and Health 18, 201-206.

Fillip, S. H., Aymanns, P. (1997): Subjektive Krankheitstheorien. In: Schwarzer, R. (Ed.): Gesundheitspsychologie. Ein Lehrbuch. Göttingen: Hogrefe, 3-21.

Flick, U. (2002): Qualitative Sozialforschung. Eine Einführung. Reinbeck bei Ham-burg: Rowohlt.

Fortune, G., Barrowclough, C., Lobban, F. (2004): Illness representations in depres-sion. British Journal of Clinical Psychology 43, 347-364.

Foulks, E.F., Persons, J. B., Merkel, R. L. (1986): The effect of patients' beliefs about their illnesses on compliance in psychotherapy. American Journal of Psychiatry 143, 340-344.

Franz, M., Lujic, C., Koch, E., Wusten, B., Yuruk, N., Gallhofer, B. (2007): Subjektive Krankheitskonzepte türkischer Migranten mit psychischen Störungen -- Besonderheiten im Vergleich zu deutschen Patienten. Psychiatrische Praxis 34, 332-338.

Freie und Hansestadt Hamburg (1998): Älter werden in der Fremde: Wohn- und Lebenssituation alterer ausländischer Hamburgerinnen und Hamburger. Sozialempirische Studie. Hamburg: Freie und Hansestadt Hamburg, Behörde für Arbeit Gesundheit und Soziales.

Freise, D. C. (2003): Teilnahme und Methodik bei Patientenbefragungen. Sankt Augustin: Asgard.

French, D.P., Senior, V., Weinman, J., Marteau, T. M. (2001): Causal attributions for heart disease: a systematic review. Psychology and Health 16, 77-98.

French, D.P., Lewin, R. J. P., Watson, N., Thompson, D. R. (2005): Do illness perceptions predict attendance at cardiac rehabilitation and quality of life following myocardial infarction? Journal of Psychosomatic Research 59, 315-322.

French, D.P., Cooper, A., Weinman, I. (2006): Illness perceptions predict attendance at cardiac rehabilitation following acute myocardial infarction: A systematic review with meta-analysis. Journal of Psychosomatic Research 61, 757-767.

Frostholm, L., Fink, P., Christensen, K. S., Toft, T., Oernboel, E., Olesen, F., Weinman, J. (2005): The patients' illness perceptions and the use of primary health care. Psychosomatic Medicine 67, 997-1005.

Fydrich, T., Sommer, G., Brähler, E. (2007): Fragebogen zur Sozialen Unterstützung (F-SozU). Manual. Göttingen: Hogrefe.

Gaskin, K., James, H. (2006): Using the Edinburgh Postnatal Depression Scale with learning disabled mothers. Community Practice 79, 392-396.

Gauchet, A., Tarquinio, C., Fischer, G. (2007): Psychosocial predictors of medication adherence among persons living with HIV. International Journal of Behavioral Medicine 14, 141-150.

Geiger, I., Razum, O. (2006): Migration. Herausforderung für die Gesundheitswissenschaften. In: Hurrelmann, K., Laaser, U., Razum, O. (Eds.): Handbuch Gesundheitswissenschaften. Weinheim: Juventa, 724-757.

Gençöz, T. (2000): Pozitif ve Negatif Duygu Ölçeği: Geçerlik ve Güvenirlik Çalışması. Türk Psikoloji Dergisi 15, 19-26.

Gerritsen, A.A., Bramsen, I., Deville, W., van Willigen, L. H., Hovens, J. E., van der Ploeg, H. M. (2004): Health and health care utilisation among asylum seekers and refugees in the Netherlands: design of a study. BMC Public Health 4, 7.

Giardini, A., Majani, G., Pierobon, A., Gremigni, P., Catapano, I. (2007): Contributo alla validazione italiana dell'IPQ-R [Contribution to the Italian validation of the IPQ-R]. Giornale Italiano di Medicina del Lavoro ed Ergonomia 29, A64-A74.

Glanz, K., Rimer, B. K., Lewis, F. M. (2002): Health behavior and health education. Theory, research, and practice. San Francisco: Jossey-Bass.

Gosciniak, H.-T. (1997): Islamische Patienten und das religiöse Fasten: Compliance versus Glauben. Deutsches Ärzteblatt 94, A-87 / B-71 / C-67.

Greenstreet, W. (2006a): From spirituality to coping strategy: making sense of chronic illness. British Journal of Nursing 15, 938-942.

Greenstreet, W. (2006b): Integrating spirituality in health and social care. Perspectives and practical approaches. Oxford: Radcliffe Medical.

Groves, R.M., Cialdini, R. B., Couper, M. P. (1992): Understanding the decision to participate in a survey. Public Opinion Quarterly 56, 475-495.

Guillemin, F., Bombardier, C., Beaton, D. (1993): Cross-cultural adaptation of health-related quality of life measures: literature review and proposed guidelines. Journal of Clinical Epidemiology 46, 1417-1432.

Hagan, N.A., Botti, M. A., Watts, R. J. (2007): Financial, family, and social factors impacting on cardiac rehabilitation attendance. Heart and Lung 36, 105-113.

Hagger, M.S., Orbell, S. (2003): A meta-analytic review of the common-sense model of illness representations. Psychology and Health 18, 141-184.

Hagger, M.S., Orbell, S. (2005): A confirmatory factor analysis of the revised illness perception questionnaire (IPQ-R) in a cervical screening context. Psychology and Health 20, 161-173.

Halligan, S.L., Cooper, P. J., Healy, S. J., Murray, L. (2007): The attribution of hostile intent in mothers, fathers and their children. Journal of Abnormal Child Psychology 35, 594-604.

Hampson, S. E. (1997): Illness representations and the self-management. In: Petrie, K.J., Weinman, J. (Eds.): Perception of health and illness. Amsterdam: Harwood, 323-347.

Hanna, L., Hunt, S., Bhopal, R. (2008): Insights from research on cross-cultural validation of health-related questionnaires. Current Sociology 56, 115-131.

Harkness, J. (1998): Cross-cultural survey equivalence. Mannheim: ZUMA.

Hedges, L. V., Olkin, I. (1985): Statistical methods for meta-analysis. Orlando: Academic.

Heider, F. (1958): The psychology of interpersonal relations. New York: Wiley.

Heijmans, M. (1999): The role of patients' illness representations in coping and functioning with Addison's disease. British Journal of Health Psychology 4, 137-149.

Helder, D.I., Kaptein, A. A., Van Kempen, G. M., Weinman, J., Van Houwelingen, J. C., Roos, R. A. (2002): Living with Huntington's disease: illness perceptions, coping mechanisms, and spouses' quality of life. International Journal of Behavioral Medicine 9, 37-52.

Helman, C. (2000): Culture, health, and illness. Oxford: Butterworth-Heinemann.

Herdman, M., Fox-Rushby, J., Badia, X. (1997): "Equivalence" and the translation of and adaptation of health-related quality of life questionnaires. Quality of Life Research 6, 237-247.

Herdman, M., Fox-Rushby, J., Badia, X. (1998): A model of equivalence in the cultural adaption of HRQoL instruments. Quality of Life Research 7, 323-335.

Higgins, R.O., Murphy, B. M., Goble, A. J., Le Grande, M. R., Elliott, P. C., Worcester, M. U. (2008): Cardiac rehabilitation program attendance after coronary artery bypass surgery: overcoming the barriers. Medical Journal of Australia 188, 712-714.

Hinnenkamp, V. (2002): Deutsch-türkisches Code-Mixing und Fragen der Hybridität. In: Hartung, W., Shethar, A. (Eds.): Kulturen und ihre Sprachen. Die Wahrnehmung anders Sprechender und ihr Selbstverständnis. Berlin: trafo verlag, 123-143.

Hinton, P. R. (2004): Statistics explained. London: Routledge.

Hirani, S.P., Newman, S. P. (2005): Patients' beliefs about their cardiovascular disease. Heart 91, 1235-1239.

Hoffmeyer-Zlotnik, J. H. P. (1985): Möglichkeiten und Grenzen der Datenerhebung bei Arbeitsmigranten. In: Sievering, U.O. (Ed.): Methodenprobleme der Datenerhebung. Frankfurt/Main: 5-24.

Holtby, R., Razmjou, H. (2005): Measurement properties of the Western Ontario rotator cuff outcome measure: a preliminary report. Journal of Shoulder and Elbow Surgery 14, 506-510.

Horne, R. (1997): Representations of medication and treatment: Advances in theory and measurement. In: Petrie, K.J., Weinman, J. (Eds.): Perception of health and illness. Amsterdam: Harwood, 155-188.

Horne, R., Weinman, J. (1999): Patients' beliefs about prescribed medicines and their role in adherence to treatment in chronic physical illness. Journal of Psychosomatic Research 47, 555-567.

Horne, R., Weinman, J., Hankins, M. (1999): The Beliefs About Medicines Questionnaire: The development and evaluation of a new method for assessing the cognitive representation of medication. Psychology and Health 1-24.

Horne, R. (1999): Patients' beliefs about treatment: The hidden determinant of treatment outcome? Journal of Psychosomatic Research 47, 491-495.

Hu, L., Bentler, P. M. (1999): Cutoff criteria for fit indexes for in covariance structure analysis: Conventional criteria versus new alternatives. Structural Equation Modeling 6, 1-55.

Huisman, M. (2000): Imputation of missing item responses: Some simple techniques. Quality and Quantity 34, 331-351.

Hunsley, J., Meyer, G. J. (2003): The incremental validity of psychological testing and assessment: Conceptual, methodological, and statistical issues. Psychological Assessment 15, 446-455.

Hunt, S.M., Bhopal, R. (2004): Self report in clinical and epidemiological studies with non-English speakers: The challenge of language and culture. Journal of Epidemiology and Community Health 58, 618-622.

Hurrelmann, K. (2003): Gesundheitssoziologie. Eine Einführung in sozialwissenschaftliche Theorien von Krankheitsprävention und Gesundheitsförderung. Weinheim/München: Juventa.

Ismail, H., Wright, J., Rhodes, P., Small, N. (2005): Religious beliefs about causes and treatment of epilepsy. British Journal of General Practice 55, 26-31.

James, D. (1999): Role of patients' perceptions on adherence to medicines and response to symptoms in MI. PhD thesis. University of Brighton.

Janz, N. K., Champion, V. L., Stretcher, V. J. (2002): The Health Belief Model. In: Glanz, K., Rimer, B.K., Lewis, F.M. (Eds.): Health behavior and health education. Theory, research, and practice. San Francisco: Jossey-Bass, 45-66.

Johns, G. (1994): How often were you absent--A review of the use of self-reported absence data. Journal of Applied Psychology 79, 574-591.

Johnson, T. P., Vijver, F. J. R. v. d. (2003): Social desirability in cross-cultural research. In: Harkness, J.A., Vijver, F.J.R.v.d., Mohler, P.P. (Eds.): Cross-cultural survey methods. Hoboken: Wiley, 195-204.

Kaiser, H.F., Rice, J. (1974): Little jiffy, mark IV. Educational and Psychological Measurement 34, 111-117.

Karanci, A.N. (1986): Causal attributions for psychological illness among Turkish psychiatric in-patients and their relationships with hope. International Journal of Social Psychiatry 32, 3-12.

Karanci, A.N. (1993): Causal attributions for illness among Turkish psychiatric outpatients and differences between diagnostic groups. Social Psychiatry and Psychiatric Epidemiology 28, 292-295.

Kärner, A. (2004): Patients' and Spouses' Perspectives on Coronary Heart Disease and its Treatment. PhD Thesis. Linköping University.

Kerns, R.D., Turk, D. C., Rudy, T. E. (1985): The West Haven-Yale Multidimensional Pain Inventory (WHYMPI). Pain 23, 345-356.

Kerswill, P. (1994): Dialects converging rural speech in urban Norway. Oxford: Clarendon Press.

King, W. (2005): Religion. In: Jones, L. (Ed.): Encyclopedia of Religion. Detroit: Macmillan Reference, 7692-7701.

Kleinman, A. (1980): Patients and healers in the context of culture. An exploration of the borderland between anthropology, medicine, and psychiatry. Berkeley: University of California Press.

Kline, P. (2000): A psychometrics primer. London: Free Association Books.

Kline, R. B. (2005): Principles and practice of structural equation modeling. New York: Guilford Press.

Kocaman, N., Özkan, M., Armay, Z., Özkan, S. (2007): Hastalık Algısı Ölçeğinin Türkçe uyarlamasının geçerlilik ve güvenilirlik çalışması [Reliability and validity study of the Turkish adaptation of the revised Illness Perception Questionnaire]. Anadolu Psikiyatri Dergisi 8, 271-280.

Koçyiğit, H., Aydemir, Ö., Fiek, G., ve ark (1999): Kisa Form (KF-36)'nin Türkçe versiyonunun güvenirlilii ve geçerlilii [Validity and reliability of Turkish version of Short form 36: A study of a patients with romatoid disorder]. Iaç ve Tedavi Dergisi 12, 102-106.

Kofahl, C. (2008): Gesundheitliche Selbsthilfe bei Menschen mit Migrationshintergrund. Public Health Forum 15, 23e1-23e3.

Koochek, A., Montazeri, A., Johansson, S. E., Sundquist, J. (2007): Health-related quality of life and migration: a cross-sectional study on elderly Iranians in Sweden. Health and Quality of Life Outcomes 5, 60.

Kubinger, D. (2005): Einige Gedanken zur Globalisierung aus Sicht der Psychologischen Diagnostik. Psychologie in Österreich 25, 58-62.

Lancaster, G.A., Dodd, S., Williamson, P. R. (2004): Design and analysis of pilot studies: recommendations for good practice. Journal of Evaluation in Clinical Practice 10, 307-312.

Lanteri-Minet, M., Massiou, H., Nachit-Ouinekh, F., Lucas, C., Pradalier, A., Radat, F., Mercier, F., El, H. A. (2007): The GRIM2005 study of migraine consultation in France I. Determinants of consultation for migraine headache in France. Cephalalgia 27, 1386-1397.

Laube, H., Bayraktar, Y., Gökce, A., Akinci, Z., Erkal, Z., Bödeker, R. H., Bilgin, Y. (2001): Zur Diabeteshäufigkeit unter türkischen Migranten in Deutschland. Diabetes und Stoffwechsel 10, 57.

Lawshe, C.H. (1975): A quantitative approach to content validity. Personnel Psychology 28, 563-557.

Lessler, J.T., O'Reilly, J. M. (1997): Mode of interview and reporting of sensitive issues: design and implementation of audio computer-assisted self-interviewing. NIDA Research Monograph 167, 366-382.

Leventhal, H., Meyer, D., Nerenez, D. (1980): The common sense representation of illness danger. In: Rachman, S. (Ed.): Contributions to medical psychology. Oxford: Pergamon Press, 7-30.

Leventhal, H., Diefenbach, M. A., Leventhal, E. A. (1992): Illness cognition: using common sense to understand treatment adherence and affect cognition interactions. Cognitive Therapy and Research 16, 143-163.

Leventhal, H., Leventhal, E. A., Cameron, L. D. (2001): Representations, procedures and affect in illness self-regulation: A perceptual-cognitive model. In: Baum, A., Revenson, T.A., Singer, J.E. (Eds.): Handbook of Health Psychology. Mahwah: Lawrence Erlbaum Associates Publishers, 19-47.

Leventhal, H., Brisette, L., Leventhal, E. A. (2003): The common-sense model of self-regulation of health and illness. In: Cameron, L.D., Leventhal, H. (Eds.): The self-regulation of health and illness behaviour. New York: Routledge, 42-65.

Lewin, R.J.P. (1999): Return to work after MI, the roles of depression, health beliefs and rehabilitation. International Journal of Cardiology 72, 49-51.

Liang, M.H. (2000): Longitudinal construct validity: establishment of clinical meaning in patient evaluative instruments. Medical Care 38, II84-90.

Lienert, G. A. (1989): Testaufbau und Testanalyse. München: Psychologie Verlags Union.

Lip, G.Y., Kamath, S., Jafri, M., Mohammed, A., Bareford, D. (2002): Ethnic differences in patient perceptions of atrial fibrillation and anticoagulation therapy: the West Birmingham Atrial Fibrillation Project. Stroke 33, 238-242.

Lobban, F., Barrowclough, C., Jones, S. (2005a): Assessing cognitive representations of mental health problems. I. The illness perception questionnaire for schizophrenia. British Journal of Clinical Psychology 44, 147-162.

Lobban, F., Barrowclough, C., Jones, S. (2005b): Assessing cognitive representations of mental health problems. II. The illness perception questionnaire for schizophrenia: Relatives' version. British Journal of Clinical Psychology 44, 163-179.

Lubkin, I. M., Larsen, P. D. (2005): What is chronicity? In: Lubkin, I.M., Larsen, P.D. (Eds.): Chronic illness: Impact and interventions. Sudbury: Jones and Bartlett, 1-24.

MacCallum, R.C., Widaman, K. F., Zhang, S., Hong, S. (1999): Sample size in factor analysis. Psychological Methods 84-99.

Machleidt, W., Behrens, K., Calliess, I. T. (2007): Integration von Migranten in die psychiatrisch-psychotherapeutische Versorgung in Deutschland. Psychiatrische Praxis 34, 331.

MacInnes, J.D. (2005): The illness perceptions of women following acute myocardial infarction: implications for behaviour change and attendance at cardiac rehabilitation. Women and Health 42, 105-121.

Maddox, G.L., Douglass, E. B. (1973): Self-assessment of health: a longitudinal study of elderly subjects. Journal of Health and Social Behavior 14, 87-93.

Maier, C., Razum, O., Schott, T. (2008): Migration und rehabilitative Versorgung in Deutschland - Inanspruchnahme von Leistungen der medizinischen Rehabilitation und Rehabilitationserfolg bei Personen mit türkischem Migrationshintergrund. Köln: Deutscher Ärzte Verlag.

Mangalam, J. J., Morgan, C. (1968): Human migration a guide to migration literature in English, 1955-1962. Lexington: University of Kentucky Press.

Marcos, Y.Q., Cantero, M. C., Escobar, C. R., Acosta, G. P. (2007): Illness perception in eating disorders and psychosocial adaptation. European Eating Disorders Review 15, 373-384.

Marsh, H.W., Hau, K. T., Balla, J. R., Grayson, D. (1998): Is more ever too much? The number of indicators per factor in confirmatory factor analysis. Multivariate Behavioral Research 33, 181-220.

Mathers, C. D., Lopez, A. D., Murray, C. J. L. (2006): The burden of disease and mortality by condition: Data, methods, and results for 2001. In: Lopez, A.D., Mathers, C.D., Ezzati, M., Jamison, D.T., Murray, C.J.L. (Eds.): Global burden of disease and risk factors. Washington, D.C: The International Bank for Reconstruction and Development / The World Bank, 45-240.

Maurer, T.J., Pierce, H. R. (1998): A comparison of Likert scale and traditional measures of self-efficacy. Journal of Applied Psychology 83, 329.

Mayring, P. (2000): Qualitative content analysis. Forum: Qualitative Social Research 1, Art. 20.

Mayring, P. (2001): Kombination und Integration qualitativer und quantitativer Analyse. Forum Qualitative Sozialforschung / Forum: Qualitative Social Research, 2(1). [Online] URL: http://www.qualitative-research.net/fqs-texte/1-01/1-01mayring-d.htm (Accessed: Apr. 01,2010)

Meraviglia, M.G. (1999): Critical analysis of spirituality and its empirical indicators. Journal of Holistic Nursing 17, 18-33.

Mesquita, B., Frijda, N. H. (1992): Cultural variations in emotions: a review. Psychological Bulletin 112, 179-204.

Minas, H., Klimidis, S., Tuncer, C. (2007): Illness causal beliefs in Turkish immigrants. BMC Psychiatry 7.

Montaño, D. E., Kasprzyk, D. (2002): The theory of reasoned action and the theory of planned behavior. In: Glanz, K., Rimer, B.K., Lewis, F.M. (Eds.): Health behavior and health education. Theory, research, and practice. San Francisco: Jossey-Bass, 67-98.

Moss-Morris, R., Weinman, I., Petrie, K. J., Horne, R., Cameron, L. D., Buick, D. (2002): The revised illness perception questionnaire (IPQ-R). Psychology and Health 17, 1-16.

Moss-Morris, R., Chalder, T. (2003): Illness perceptions and levels of disability in patients with chronic fatigue syndrome and rheumatoid arthritis. Journal of Psychosomatic Research 55, 305-308.

Mullen, P.D., Mains, D. A., Velez, R. (2008): A meta-analysis of controlled trials of cardiac patient education. Patient Education and Counseling 19, 143-162.

Munro, B. H. (2005): Statistical methods for health care research. Philadelphia: Lippincott Williams & Wilkins.

Murdock, G.P., Wilson, S. F., Frederick, V. (1978): World distribution of theories of illness. Ethnology: An International Journal of Cultural and Social Anthropology 17, 470.

Murphy, E., Kinmonth, A. L. (1995): No symptoms, no problem? Patients' understandings of non-insulin dependent diabetes. Family Practice 12, 184-192.

Münz, R., Ulrich, R. E. (2001): Migration und zukünftige Bevölkerungsentwicklung in Deutschland. In: Franz, W. (Ed.): Wirtschaftspolitische Herausforderungen an der Jahrhundertwende. Tübingen: Mohr Siebeck, 181-200.

Myers, R.E. (2003): Self-regulation and decision making about cancer screening. In: Cameron, L.D., Leventhal, H. (Eds.): The self-regulation of health and illness behaviour. London: Routledge, 297-313.

Naz, Ö. (2006): Sind turkischsprachige Mitbürgerinnen und Mitbürger schwieriger zur Teilnahme an einer Selbsthilfegruppe zu motivieren? In: Deutsche Arbeitsgemeinschaft Selbsthilfegruppen e.V. (Ed.). Gießen: Focus Verlag, 72-75.

Nickel, M., Cangoez, B., Bachler, E., Muehlbacher, M., Lojewski, N., Mueller-Rabe, N., Mitterlehner, F. O., Leiberich, P., Rother, N., Buschmann, W., Kettler, C., Pedrosa Gil, F., Lahmann, C., Egger, C., Fartacek, R., Rother, W. K., Loew, T. H., Nickel, C. (2006): Bioenergetic exercises in inpatient treatment of Turkish immigrants with chronic somatoform disorders: a randomized, controlled study. Journal of Psychosomatic Research 61, 507-513.

Nielsen, K.M., Faergeman, O., Foldspang, A., Larsen, M. L. (2008): Cardiac rehabilitation: health characteristics and socio-economic status among those who do not attend. European Journal of Public Health 18, 479-483.

O'Conner, B.P. (2000): SPSS and SAS programs for determining the number of components using parallel analysis and Velicer's MAP test. Behavior Research Methods, Instrumentation, and Computers 32, 396-402.

Osborne, J.W., Costello, A. B. (2004): Sample size and subject to item ratio in principal component analysis. Practical Assessment, Research & Evaluation 9.

Ozankan, M. (2008): Bedürfnisangepasste Behandlung älterer Migrantinnen und Migranten - Interkulturelle Öffnung der psychiatrischen Regelversorgung. In: Teschauer, W., Sürer, F. (Eds.): Diagnostik - Diagnostik und Versorgung bei türkischen Migranten in Deutschland. Beiträge des internationalen Expertengespräches vom 18. bis 20. Januar 2008 in Ingolstadt. Ingolstadt: Ingenium-Stiftung, 43-52.

Önder, S. W. (2007): We have no microbes here: Healing practices in a Turkish Black Sea village. Durkham: Carolina Academic Press.

Öztürk, O. M., Goksel, F. A. (1964): Folk treatment of mental illness in Turkey. In: Kiev, A. (Ed.): Magic, Faith and Healing. New York: The Free Press, 343-363.

Öztürk, O.M. (1965): Folk interpretation of illness in Turkey and its psychological significance. Turkish Journal of Pediatrics 7, 165-179.

Padilla, A. M. (2001): Issues in culturally appropriate assessment. In: Suzuki, L.A., Pnterotto, J.G., Meller, P.J. (Eds.): Handbook of multicultural assessment. San Francisco: Jossey-Bass, 5-27.

Pargament, K.I., Koenig, H. G., Tarakeshwar, N., Hahn, J. (2001): Religious struggle as a predictor of mortality among medically ill elderly patients: a 2-year longitudinal study. Archives of Internal Medicine 161, 1881-1885.

Paschalides, C., Wearden, A. J., Dunkerley, R., Bundy, C., Davies, R., Dickens, C. M. (2004): The associations of anxiety, depression and personal illness representations with glycaemic control and health-related quality of life in patients with type 2 diabetes mellitus. Journal of Psychosomatic Research 57, 557-564.

Patel, R.P., Taylor, S. D. (2002): Factors affecting medication adherence in hypertensive patients. The Annals of Pharmacotherapy 36, 40-45.

Pavkovic, G. (2004): Beratung für Migranten. In: Nestmann, F., Engel, F., Sickendiek, U. (Eds.): Das Handbuch der Beratung, Band 1: Disziplinen und Zugänge. Tübingen: dgvt-Verlag, 305-311.

Perneger, T.V., Burnand, B. (2005): A simple imputation algorithm reduced missing data in SF-12 health surveys. Journal of Clinical Epidemiology 58, 142-149.

Peters, M., Passchier, J. (2006): Translating instruments for cross-cultural studies in headache research. Headache 46, 82-91.

Peterson, R. A. (2000): Constructing effective questionnaires. Thousand Oaks: Sage.

Petrie, K.J., Weinman, J., Sharpe, N., Buckley, J. (1996): Role of patients' view of their illness in predicting return to work and functioning after myocardial infarction: Longitudinal study. British Medical Journal 312, 1191-1194.

Petrie, K. J., Weinman, J. (1997): Illness representation and recovery from myocardial infarction. In: Petrie, K.J., Weinman, J. (Eds.): Perceptions of health and illness. Current Research and Applications. Amsterdam: Harwood Academic Publishers, 441-461.

Petrie, K.J., Cameron, L. D., Ellis, C. J., Buick, D., Weinman, J. (2002): Changing illness perceptions after myocardial infarction: An early intervention randomized controlled trial. Psychosomatic Medicine 64, 580-586.

Petrie, K. J., Broadbent, E., Meechan, G. (2003): Self-regulatory interventions for improving the management of chronic illness. In: Cameron, L.D., Leventhal, R. (Eds.): The self-regulation of health and illness behaviour. New York: Routledge, 257-277.

Petrie, K.J., Broadbent, E., Ellis, C., Ying.J. (2005): Improving recovery following heart attacks by changing illness perceptions: A randomised trial. Psychology and Health 20 (Suppl), 212.

Pinar, R. (2005): Reliability and construct validity of the SF-36 in Turkish cancer patients. Quality of Life Research 14, 259-264.

Podsakoff, P.M., MacKenzie, S. B., Lee, J.-Y., Podsakoff, N. P. (2003): Common method biases in behavioral research: A critical review of the literature and recommended reading. Journal of Applied Psychology 88, 879-903.

Porter, A.C., Gamoran, A. (2002): Methodological advances in cross-national surveys of educational achievement. Washington: National Academic Press.

Püringer, U. (2007): Grundlagenkonzept zu Interventionen der Herz-Kreislauf-Gesundheit in Österreich. Wien. [Online] URL: http://www.fgoe.org/der-fonds/prioritaten/herz-kreislaufgesundheit/2008-10-03.8373037224/download (Accessed: Apr. 01,2010)

QualityMetric Inc. (2008): IQOLA Project SF-12v2™ Health Survey (Second version) Translations available through QualityMetric Incorporated. [Online] URL: http://www.qualitymetric.com/ (Accessed: Apr. 01,2010)

Razum, O., Geiger, I., Zeeb, H., Ronellenfitsch, U. (2004): Gesundheitsversorgung von Migranten. Deutsches Ärzteblatt 101, A2882-A2887.

Razum, O., Zeeb, H., Meesmann, U., Schenk, L., Bredehorst, M., Brzoska, P., Dercks, T., Glodny, S., Menkhaus, B., Salman, R., Saß, A.-C., Ulrich, R. (2008): Migration und Gesundheit. Berlin: Robert Koch-Institut.

Reijneveld, S.A., Westhoff, M. H., Hopman-Rock, M. (2003): Promotion of health and physical activity improves the mental health of elderly immigrants: results of a group randomised controlled trial among Turkish immigrants in the Netherlands aged 45 and over. Journal of Epidemiology and Community Health 57, 405-411.

Riley, D.L., Stewart, D. E., Grace, S. L. (2007): Continuity of cardiac care: cardiac rehabilitation participation and other correlates. International Journal of Cardiology 119, 326-333.

Ronellenfitsch, U., Razum, O. Deteriorating health satisfaction among immigrants from Eastern Europe to Germany. International Journal of Equity in Health 3 (1):4, 2004.

Ross, S., Walker, A., MacLeod, M. J. (2004): Patient compliance in hypertension: Role of illness perceptions and treatment beliefs. Journal of Human Hypertension 18, 607-613.

Rothman, A.J., Kelly, K.M., Hertel, A.W., Salovey, P. (2003): Message frames and illness representations: implications for interventions to promote and sustain healthy behavior. In: Cameron, L.D., Leventhal, H. (Eds.): The self-regulation of health and illness behaviour. London: Routledge, 278-296.

Sabit, R., Griffiths, T. L., Watkins, A. J., Evans, W., Bolton, C. E., Shale, D. J., Lewis, K. E. (2008): Predictors of poor attendance at an outpatient pulmonary rehabilitation programme. Respiratory Medicine 102, 819-824.

Sapnas, K.G., Zeller, R. A. (2002): Minimizing sample size when using exploratory factor analysis for measurement. Journal of Nursing Measurement 10, 135-154.

Schaeffer, D., Moers, M. (2003): Bewältigung chronischer Krankheit -- Aufgaben der Pflege. In: Rennen-Allhoff, B., Schaeffer, D. (Eds.): Handbuch Pflegewissenschaft. Weinheim: Juventa, 447-483.

Schaeffer, D. (2004): Der Patient als Nutzer - eine Analyse des Bewältigungs- und Nutzungshandelns im Verlauf chronischer Krankheit. Bern: Verlag Hans Huber.

Schaeffer, D. (2005): Versorgungswirklichkeit in der letzten Lebensphase: Ergebnisse einer Analyse der Nutzerperspektive. In: Ewers, M., Schaeffer, D. (Eds.): Am Ende des Lebens. Bern: Verlag Hans Huber, 69-71.

Scharloo, M., Kaptein, A. A. (1997): Measurement of illness perception in patients with chronic somatic illness: A review. In: Petrie, K.J., Weinman, J. (Eds.): Perception of health and illness. Amsterdam: Harwood, 103-154.

Scharloo, M., Kaptein, A. A., Weinman, J. A., Willems, L. N., Rooijmans, H. G. (2000): Physical and psychological correlates of functioning in patients with chronic obstructive pulmonary disease. Journal of Asthma 37, 17-29.

Schönberg, U. (1985): Probleme der inhaltlichen und sprachlichen Gestaltung standardisierter Befragungsinstrumente und deren Übersetzung in Untersuchungen über Arbeitsmigranten. In: Sievering, U.O. (Ed.): Methodenprobleme der Datenerhebung. Frankfurt/Main: 5.

Schwarzer, R., Jerusalem, M. (1995): In: Weinman, J., Wright, S., Johnston, M. (Eds.): Measures in health psychology: A user's portfolio. Causal and control beliefs. Windsor: Nfer-Nelson, 35-37.

Searle, A., Norman, P., Thompson, R., Vedhara, K. (2007): Illness representations among patients with type 2 diabetes and their partners: relationships with self-management behaviors. Journal of Psychosomatic Research 63, 175-184.

Sen, F., Goldberg, A. (1994): Türken in Deutschland. München: Beck.

Senior, V., Marteau, T. M., Weinman, J. (2004): Self-reported adherence to cholesterol-lowering medication in patients with familial hypercholesterolaemia: the role of illness perceptions. Cardiovascular Drugs and Therapy 18, 475-481.

Sherman, A.C., Pennington, J., Simonton, S., Latif, U., Arent, L., Farley, H. (2008): Determinants of participation in cancer support groups: the role of health beliefs. International Journal of Behavioral Medicine 15, 92-100.

Skinner, C.S., Siegfried, J. C., Kegler, M. C., Stretcher, V. J. (1993): The potential of computers in patient education. Patient Education and Counselling 22, 27-34.

Song, J., Belin, T. R. (2008): Choosing an appropriate number of factors in factor analysis with incomplete data. Computational Statistics & Data Analysis 52, 3560-3569.

Spallek, J., Razum, O. (2007): Gesundheit von Migranten: Defizite im Bereich der Prävention. Medizinische Klinik 102, 451-456.

Spallek, J., Razum, O. (2008): Gleich und gerecht? Erklärungsmodelle für die gesundheitliche Situation von Migrantinnen und Migranten. In: Bauer, U., Bittlingmayer, U.H., Richter, M. (Eds.): Health Inequalities. Determinanten und Mechanismen gesundheitlicher Ungleichheit. Wiesbaden: VS Verlag für Sozialwissenschaften

Spielberg, C.D., Moscoso, M.S., Brunner, T.M. (2005): Cross-cultural assessment of emotional states and personality traits. In: Hambleton, R.K., Merenda, P.F., Spielberger, C.D. (Eds.): Adapting educational and psychological tests for cross-cultural assessment. Mahwah: Lawrence Erlbaum Associates, 343-367.

SPSS Inc. (2006): SPSS for Windows 15. Chicago: SPSS Inc.

Statistisches Bundesamt (2009): Bevölkerung und Erwerbstätigkeit. Bevölkerung mit Migrationshintergrund. Ergebnisse des Mikrozensus 2007. Wiesbaden: Statistisches Bundesamt.

Stevens, S.S. (1946): On the theory of scales of measurement. Science 103, 677-680.

Stewart, A.L., Napoles-Springer, A. (2000): Health-related quality-of-life assessments in diverse population groups in the United States. Medical Care 38, II102-II124.

SVR - Sachverständigenrat für die Konzentrierte Aktion im Gesundheitswesen (2001): Bedarfsgerechtigkeit und Wirtschaftlichkeit. Band 3: Über-, Unter- und Fehlversorgung. Gutachten 2000/2001. Ausführliche Zusammenfassung. Bonn: Sachverständigenrat für die Konzentrierte Aktion im Gesundheitswesen.

Tabachnick, B. G., Fidell, L. S. (1996): Using multivariate statistics. New Jersey: Erlbaum.

Tagay, S., Zararsiz, R., Erim, Y., Dullmann, S., Schlegl, S., Brahler, E., Senf, W. (2008): Traumatische Ereignisse und Posttraumatische Belastungsstörung bei türkischsprachigen Patienten in der Primärversorgung. Psychotherapie, Psychosomatik, medizinische Psychologie 58, 155-161.

Teddlie, C., Tashakkori, A. (2003): Major issues and controversies in the use of mixed methods in the social and behavioral sciences. In: Tashakkori, A., Teddlie, C. (Eds.): Handbook of mixed methods in social & behavioral research. Thousand Oaks, CA: Sage, 3-50.

Tellegen, A. (1985): Structures of mood and personality and their relevance to assessing anxiety, with an emphasis on self-report. In: Tuma, A.H., Maser, J.D. (Eds.): Anxiety and the Anxiety disorders. Hilssdale: Erlbaum, 681-706.

Thielmann, J. (2008): Varied forms of muslim religiousness in Germany. In: Bertelsmann Stiftung (Ed.): Religion Monitor 2008. Muslim religiousness in Germany. Overview of religious attitudes and practices. Gütersloh: Bertelsmann Stiftung, 13-21.

Thomas, L. (1974): Commentary: The future impact of science and technology on medicine. Bioscience 24, 95-104.

Thomson ResearchSoft (2005): Reference Manager Version 11. Berkeley.

Tilli, K. (1989): Psychosomatische Erkrankungen türkischer Frauen in der Bundesrepublik Deutschland. Ätiologische Konzepte türkischer Frauen und ihre Bedeutung für die Arzt-Patienten-Beziehung. In: Söllner, W., Wesiak, W., Wurm, B. (Eds.): Soziopsychosomatik. Berlin: Springer, 222-228.

Trotter (1988): Orientation to multicultural health care in migrant health programs. Austin: National Migrant Referral Project.

Turk, D.C., Rudy, T. E., Salovey, P. (1986): Implicit models of illness. Journal of Behavioral Medicine 9, 453-474.

Ucar, A. (1996): Benachteiligt: Ausländische Kinder in der deutschen Sonderschule. Hohengehren: Schneider Verlag.

University of Wollongong (2005): Instrument review: SF-12 Health Survey (Version 1.0). [Online] URL: http://chsd.uow.edu.au/ahoc/documents/sf12review.pdf (Accessed: Apr. 01,2010)

Van de Vijver, F., Hambleton, R. K. (1996): Translating Tests: Some Practical Guidelines. European Psychologist 1, 89-99.

Van de Vijver, F. J. R. (2001): The evolution of cross-cultural research methods. In: Matsumoto, D. (Ed.): The handbook of culture and psychology. New York: Oxford University Press, 77-97.

Vázquez, M.B., Bermejo Alegria, R. M., Garcia Ayala, M. D. (2005): Estructura factorial de la versión española del Revised Illness Perception Questionnaire en una muestra de hipertensos. Psicothema 17, 318-324.

Verres, R. (1986): Krebs und Angst. Subjektive Theorien von Laien über Entstehung, Vorsorge, Früherkennung, Behandlung und die psychosozialen Folgen von Krebserkrankungen. Berlin: Springer.

Voerman, B., Visser, A., Fischer, M., Garssen, B., van Andel, G., Bensing, J. (2007): Determinants of participation in social support groups for prostate cancer patients. Psycho-Oncology 16, 1092-1099.

Wallston, K. A., Wallston, B. S. (1982): Who is responsible for your health? The construct of Health Locus of Control. In: Sanders, G., Suls, J. (Eds.): Social Psychology of Health and Illness. Hillsdale: Lawrence Erlbaum Associates, 65-95.

Walsh, J.C., Lynch, M., Murphy, A. W., Daly, K. (2004): Factors influencing the decision to seek treatment for symptoms of acute myocardial infarction: an evaluation of the Self-Regulatory Model of illness behaviour. Journal of Psychosomatic Research 56, 67-73.

Ware, J., Jr., Kosinski, M., Keller, S. D. (1995): SF-12: How to score the SF-12 Physical and Mental Health Summary Scales. Boston, MA: The Health Institute, New England Medical Center.

Ware, J., Jr., Kosinski, M., Keller, S. D. (1996): A 12-Item Short-Form Health Survey: construction of scales and preliminary tests of reliability and validity. Medical Care 34, 220-233.

Ware, J., Jr., Kosinski, M., Dewey, J. E. (2000): How to Score Version Two of the SF-36 Health Survey. Lincoln: QualityMetric, Inc.

Ware, J., Jr., Kosinski, M., Dewey, J. E., Gandek, B. (2001): How to score and interpret single-item health status measures: A manual for users of the SF-8 Health Survey. Lincoln: QualityMetric, Inc.

Ware, J., Jr. (2003): SF-36® Health Survey update. Lincoln: QualityMetric Incorporated. [Online] URL: http://www.sf-36.org/tools/SF36.shtml (Accessed: Apr. 01,2010)

Ware, J.E., Jr., Sherbourne, C. D. (1992): The MOS 36-item short-form health survey (SF-36). I. Conceptual framework and item selection. Medical Care 30, 473-483.

Watson, D., Clark, L. A., Tellegen, A. (1988): Development and validation of brief measures of positive and negative affect: the PANAS scales. Journal of Personality and Social Psychology 54, 1063-1070.

Weber, M. (1978): Economy and society : an outline of interpretive sociology. Wirtschaft und Gesellschaft. English. Berkeley: University of California Press.

Weilandt, C., Altenhofen, L. (1997): Gesundheit und gesundheitliche Versorgung von Migranten. In: Weber, I. (Ed.): Gesundheit sozialer Randgruppen: gesundheitliche Probleme gesellschaftlich benachteiligter Gruppen und deren Versorgung. Stuttgart: Enke, 76-96.

Weinman, J., Petrie, K. J., Moss-Morris, R., Horne, R. (1996): The Illness Perception Questionnaire: A new method for assessing the cognitive representation of illness. Psychology and Health 11, 431-445.

Weinman, J., Petrie, K. J., Sharpe, N., Walker, S. (2000): Causal attributions in patients and spouses following a heart attack and subsequent lifestyle changes. British Journal of Health Psychology 5, 263-273.

White, J.B. (1997): Turks in the new Germany. American Anthropologist 99, 754-769.

Whitmarsh, A., Koutantji, M., Sidell, K. (2003): Illness perceptions, mood and coping in predicting attendance at cardiac rehabilitation. British Journal of Health Psychology 8, 209-221.

WHO (1973): Report of International Pilot Study for Schizophrenia. Geneva: World Health Organization.

WHO (2005): Preventing chronic diseases. A vital investment. Geneva.

WHO Regional Committee for Europe (2006): Gaining Health. The European Strategy for the Prevention and Control of Noncommunicable Diseases. [Online] URL: http://www.euro.who.int/document/rc56/edoc08.pdf (Accessed: Apr. 01,2010)

Wright, D.L., Aquilino, W. S., Supple, A. J. (1998): A comparison of computer-assisted and paper-and-pencil self-administered questionnaires in a survey on smoking alcohol, and drug use. Public Opinion Quarterly 62, 623-632.

Wunn, I. (2006): Muslimische Patienten. Chancen und Grenzen religionsspezifischer Pflege. Stuttgart: Kohlhammer.

Yeşilay A., Schwarzer R., Jerusalem M. (no date): Genelleştirilmiş özyetki beklentisi. [Online] URL: http://userpage.fu-berlin.de/~health/turk.htm (Accessed Apr. 01, 2010)

Yildirim-Fahlbusch, Y. (2003): Kulturelle Missverständnisse. Die Beziehung zwischen deutschen Ärzten und ihren türkischen Patienten gestaltet sich oft schwierig. Sprachprobleme sind dabei nur die Spitze des Eisbergs. Deutsches Ärzteblatt 100, A-1179 / B-993 / C-928.

Yohannes, A.M., Yalfani, A., Doherty, P., Bundy, C. (2007): Predictors of drop-out from an outpatient cardiac rehabilitation programme. Clinical Rehabilitation 21, 222-229.

Zeeb, H., Kutschmann, M., Razum, O. (2005): Gesundheitszufriedenheit alternder Migranten eine Analyse mit Daten des Sozioökonomischen Panels (SOEP). 8. lögd-Jahrestagung "Demografische Alterung und Gesundheit" am 25./26.3. 2005. [Online] URL: http://www.loegd.nrw.de/1pdf_dokumente/1_allgemeine-dienste/tagungen/050408bielefeld_8-oegd-tagung/zeeb_kutschmann_razum_gesundheitszufriedenheit.mht (Accessed: Apr. 01,2010)

Appendix A: Additional tables and figures

A.1   Additional tables

Study	Country	Design	Instrument	Main results regarding illness beliefs and attendance at cardiac I rehabilitation
Petrie et al. (1996)	NZ	Cross-sectional, group comparison, hospital survey, post-MI patients, n=128.	IPQ	Significant associations with attendance: - Strong belief about **controllability** (g=0.40) *No association with identity and timeline*
Cooper et al. (1999)	UK	Cross-sectional, group comparison, hospital survey, patients after MI or Bypass operation, n=152.	IPQ	Significant associations with attendance: - Strong beliefs about **controllability** (g=0.45) - **Causal attribution** (behavior, life style) (g=0.63) *No association with timeline and consequences*
James (1999)	UK	Cross-sectional, group comparison, hospital survey, patients after MI or Bypass operation, n=130.	IPQ	*No significant association*
Petrie et al. (2002)	NZ	Cross-sectional, group comparison, survey short before discharge from hospital, post-MI patients, n=62.	IPQ	Strong association with attendance, but non-significant. Could be attributable to low sample size. - Weak **identity** (g=-0.4) - **Timeline** (belief about long duration) (g=-0.73) - Strong beliefs about **controllability** (g=0.67) - Weak beliefs about **consequences** (g=-0.70)
Whitmarsh et al. (2003)	UK	Cross-sectional, group comparison, survey short before discharge from hospital, post-MI patients, n=93.	IPQ	Significant associations with attendance: - Strong **identity** (g=0.77) - Strong beliefs about **consequences** (g=0.67) *No association with timeline, controllability, causal attributions*
Cooper (2004)	UK	Cross-sectional, group comparison, hospital survey, post-MI patients, n=117.	IPQ-R	*No significant association*
MacInnes (2005)	UK	Qualitative design, semi-structured interviews. 3 months post-MI, female patients, n=10.		Attendance was associated with strong beliefs about **controllability** and the feeling of knowing the cause of one's illness.
Petrie et al. (2005)	NZ	Cross-sectional, group comparison, survey short before discharge from hospital, post-MI patients, n=85	Brief IPQ	*No significant association*
French et al. (2005)	UK	Cross-sectional, group comparison, survey 24h after admission to hospital, post-MI patients, n=194.	IPQ	*No significant association*
Yohannes et al. (2007)	UK	Cross-sectional, group comparison, participants of a rehabilitation program, n=147, outcome examined: drop-out.	IPQ-R	Significant associations with continued attendance, bivariate: - Strong beliefs about **consequences** (g=0.70) - Weak belief about **personal controllability** (g=-0.46) - Strong belief about **treatment controllability** (g=0.37) - Weak **identity** (g=-0.40) - Strong beliefs about **timeline (acute/chronic)** (g=0.40) *No association with emotional representations and illness coherence* Significant associations with continued attendance, bivariate: - Strong beliefs about **consequences** (OR=1.64) - Weak belief about **personal controllability** (OR=0.5) - Strong belief about **treatment controllability** (OR=1.96)

Note. IPQ(-R): Illness Perception Questionnaire (revised); MI: myocardial infarction

Tab. A 1: Overview of studies on the role of illness beliefs in attendance at cardiac rehabilitation (Source: Own illustration)

Study	Country	Design	Instrument	Main results regarding illness beliefs and adherence
Patel und Tylor (2002)	USA	Cross-sectional, group comparison, survey in hypertension clinic, hypertensive patients, n=128.	self-made	Significant associations with adherence: - Weak beliefs about **controllability** (Kendalls τ=-0.31) *No significant association with causal attributions*
Brewer et al. (2002)	USA	Cross-sectional, group comparison, survey in a general clinic, patients hypercholesterinaemia, n=169.	IPQ	Significant associations with adherence - strong beliefs about **consequences** (standardized beta=0.28) *No significant association with causal attributions, timeline, identity, controllability.*
Senior et al. (2004)	UK	Cross-sectional, group comparison, therapy against high cholesterol levels n=336	Instrument for assessing beliefs about cardiovascular diseases	Significant associations with adherence (descriptive): - Weak beliefs about **consequences** (g=-0.65). - Strong beliefs about **controllability** (g=0.33) - Strong **causal attributions** (heredity g=0.34) Significant associations with adherence (multivariate): - Strong **causal attributions** (heredity OR=1.31)
Ross et al. (2004)	UK	Cross-sectional, group comparison, survey in hypertension clinic, hypertensive patients, n=493.	IPQ-R	Significant associations with adherence (descriptive): - Weak beliefs about **personal controllability** (g=-0.38) - Strong beliefs about **treatment controllability** (g=0.26) - Weak **emotional representations** (g=-0.31) - Weak beliefs about **consequences** (g=-0.28) *No significant association with coherence, identity, timeline, causal attributions.* Significant associations with adherence (multivariate): - Weak **emotional representations** (OR=0.65) - Weak beliefs about **personal controllability** (OR=0.59)
Byrne et al. (2005)	IRL	Cross-sectional, group comparison, pharmacotherapy for secondary prevention of cardiovascular diseases, patients recruited from 35 general practitioner offices, n=1611	IPQ-R	Significant associations with adherence (descriptive): - strong beliefs about duration of illness (r=0.1) *No significant association with coherence, identity, causal attributions, consequences, emotional representations, controllability* Significant associations with adherence (multivariate) - *No significant associations*

Note. IPQ(-R): Illness Perception Questionnaire (revised)

Tab. A 2: Overview of studies on the role of illness beliefs in adherence to long-term therapies (Source: Own illustration)

	1	2	3	4	5	6	7	8	9	10	11	12	13	14	15	16	17	18	19	20	21	22	23	24	25	26	27	28	29	30	31	32	33	34	35	36	37	38
C1	1
C2	-.1	1
C3	-.1	.7	1
C4	.4	-.1	-.1	1
C5	.0	.5	.4	.4	1
C6	.0	.3	.2	.0	.4	1
C7	-.1	.3	.3	-.1	.5	.5	1
C8	-.1	-.1	-.2	.3	.2	.2	.4	1
C9	-.1	-.3	-.2	.1	-.1	.3	.0	.0	1
C10	-.1	-.2	-.1	.0	.0	.0	.0	-.1	.0	1
C11	.0	-.2	-.2	.0	-.2	.0	-.3	-.1	-.1	.5	1
C12	-.1	-.2	-.2	.1	-.1	.2	.0	-.2	-.1	-.2	.1	1
C13	.0	-.1	-.1	.1	.0	-.1	.3	.3	.0	-.1	-.2	.2	1
C14	-.1	-.2	-.2	-.1	-.3	-.1	.4	.2	-.3	-.2	-.2	-.3	.5	1
C15	.0	-.1	-.1	.0	-.2	-.3	.3	.0	-.1	-.3	-.3	-.2	.3	.6	1
C16	-.1	-.1	-.1	-.3	.0	.2	.3	.2	-.1	.0	-.1	.0	.4	.2	.2	1
C17	-.1	.3	.0	-.1	.4	.1	.1	.0	-.2	.0	.0	-.2	-.1	-.3	-.1	-.1	1
C18	-.3	.0	.0	-.3	.0	.0	.0	-.3	-.2	.0	-.1	-.1	.0	-.2	-.3	.0	-.3	1
C19	.3	-.2	-.1	.0	-.1	-.2	-.1	.4	-.3	.1	-.1	.1	.0	-.2	-.3	.3	-.2	.0	1
C20	.0	.3	.0	.0	.3	-.1	-.1	.1	-.2	.0	-.3	-.1	.0	.2	-.1	.3	-.1	-.1	-.2	1
C21	.0	-.2	-.1	-.1	.0	-.2	-.1	-.2	-.1	.0	-.1	.0	.2	-.1	.0	-.3	-.2	-.4	.4	-.1	1
C22	-.2	-.2	-.1	-.1	-.1	-.1	-.1	-.2	-.2	.0	.0	-.2	.2	.0	.0	-.1	.0	-.2	-.2	.1	-.2	1
C23	-.1	-.1	-.2	-.2	.0	-.1	.0	-.1	-.1	-.2	.2	.0	.3	.4	.3	.0	-.3	-.1	-.2	-.2	-.3	.5	1
C24	.0	-.1	.0	-.1	.0	-.1	-.3	.0	.0	.0	.0	-.2	.2	-.2	-.2	-.2	-.1	.4	.0	.2	-.1	.4	-.2	1
C25	.2	-.1	-.2	-.1	.0	.0	-.1	.0	.0	-.1	-.1	.0	-.1	.0	.0	-.1	.0	.0	.2	-.2	.2	.2	-.1	.0	1
C26	.2	-.1	.0	.0	.0	-.1	-.1	-.1	-.3	.1	-.1	.0	-.1	-.1	-.3	.2	-.1	-.2	-.2	.2	.2	-.1	-.1	.4	.5	1
C27	.1	.3	.0	-.1	-.1	.0	.0	.0	.0	.3	.0	.4	-.1	-.1	-.3	.0	-.1	.0	-.4	-.1	-.1	-.1	-.1	-.1	-.5	.4	1
C28	.1	-.1	-.1	-.2	.0	-.1	.3	-.2	.1	-.1	-.1	-.2	.1	.0	.0	.0	-.2	.0	.1	-.2	-.1	-.2	.0	.3	.0	.2	.4	1
C29	-.1	.0	.1	.1	-.1	-.1	.0	-.1	-.3	.1	.2	.0	.3	.0	.3	.0	.3	.2	.4	.3	.3	.3	.0	-.2	.0	-.1	.0	-.1	1
C30	-.2	-.2	-.2	-.1	-.2	.0	-.1	-.2	-.1	-.2	-.1	-.3	-.1	.2	.2	.1	-.1	-.3	.2	.0	-.1	.2	-.1	.4	.0	-.3	-.2	.2	-.2	1
C31	-.1	-.1	-.1	-.1	-.1	-.1	.0	-.1	-.1	.0	.5	.0	.0	-.1	.0	.0	.0	-.2	-.1	-.1	.0	.3	-.2	-.1	-.2	.4	.2	-.1	-.1	.2	1
C32	.0	-.2	-.1	-.1	-.3	-.2	.5	.5	.0	-.1	.0	-.2	.3	.3	-.2	-.2	.1	-.3	-.2	-.2	-.2	-.1	.3	.0	.0	-.1	.0	.0	-.1	-.1	.0	1
C33	-.1	.0	-.1	.0	-.2	-.4	-.2	-.2	-.1	-.2	.3	.3	.2	.4	.0	.0	-.1	-.2	-.2	-.2	.0	-.4	-.1	-.2	.0	-.2	.0	.0	-.4	-.1	-.1	-.2	1
C34	-.1	.0	-.1	-.1	-.1	-.1	.3	.1	-.2	.0	.2	-.2	.3	.3	.4	.2	.4	-.1	-.2	.1	-.1	-.1	-.1	-.1	-.0	-.4	-.1	-.3	.4	-.3	.0	-.1	.2	1
C35	-.1	-.1	.2	-.1	.2	.0	.1	-.2	.0	-.3	.1	.3	-.1	-.2	-.3	-.1	-.3	.0	-.1	.5	-.3	.2	-.2	-.2	.2	-.3	-.4	-.1	.3	-.2	.4	-.1	.2	.3	1
C36	-.1	.0	.0	-.1	-.1	-.1	-.1	-.3	.1	.0	.0	-.1	.2	.3	.0	.0	-.2	.2	.0	-.1	-.1	.2	.2	-.3	.2	-.2	-.1	.3	-.2	-.2	-.2	-.1	.3	.2	.6	1
C37	-.1	-.1	-.1	-.1	-.1	.3	.0	.0	-.1	.0	.0	-.2	-.1	-.2	-.1	.0	.0	.4	-.3	-.1	-.1	-.1	-.4	.0	-.2	-.1	.1	.2	-.2	-.2	.3	-.2	-.2	-.1	-.2	-.3	1
C38	-.2	-.1	-.2	-.1	-.4	-.1	-.1	-.4	-.4	.4	.4	.1	.3	.3	.3	.1	-.1	-.2	.2	-.4	-.2	.4	.5	.0	.3	.5	.6	.1	-.1	.0	.2	-.1	.5	.8	.4	.3	-.5	.8

Tab. A 3: Correlation matrix of IPQ-R part II items (Source: Own data)

Tab. A 4: Anti-image correlation matrix and measures of sample adequacy of the IPQ-R part II (Source: Own data)

	D1	D2	D3	D4	D5	D6	D7	D8	D9	D10	D11	D12	D13	D14	D15	D16	D17	D18	D19
D1		.22	.01	.16	.16	.28*	.30*	.17	.38*	.46*	.51*	.29*	.30*	.16	.09	.02	.07	.30*	-.13
D2			.10	.33*	.07	-.08	.08	.17	.07	.02	.00	.24*	-.07	.09	.06	.00	-.09	-.04	-.16
D3				.27*	.17	.26*	.39*	.25*	.15	.22	.00	.02	.01	-.34*	.17	.28*	.15	-.05	.06
D4					.05	.02	.23	.29*	.15	.19	-.01	.34*	.13	-.14	.15	.05	.00	.12	-.13
D5						.46*	.10	.21	.31*	.30*	.13	.33*	.07	.19	.00	.13	.23*	.21	.09
D6							.41	.37*	.33*	.51*	.44*	.24*	.29*	-.04	.04	.32*	.35*	.28*	.02
D7								.43*	.43*	.40*	.27*	.17	.27*	-.03	.35*	.37*	.18	.18	-.19
D8									.40*	.37*	.30*	.32*	.13	.06	.22	.23	.29*	.07	-.03
D9										.45*	.32*	.38*	.18	.07	.26*	.21	.26*	.28*	.14
D10											.42*	.63*	.39*	.08	.25*	.27*	.32*	.40*	.10
D11												.30*	.31*	.03	.05	.26*	.19	.49*	.01
D12													.24*	.14	.03	.00	.25*	.34*	.01
D13														.29*	.18	.24*	.16	.35*	.03
D14															.00	.01	.03	.02	.10
D15																.42*	.26*	.01	.18
D16																	.50*	.03	.29*
D17																		.20	.21
D18																			.06
D19																			

Tab. A 5: Correlation matrix of IPQ-R part III items on causal attributions (Source: Own data)

	D1	D2	D3	D4	D5	D6	D7	D8	D9	D10	D11	D12	D13	D14	D15	D16	D17	D18	D19
D1	.60																		
D2	-.27	.47																	
D3	.21	-.21	.44																
D4	-.21	-.12	-.25	.44															
D5	-.11	-.02	-.26	.14	.56														
D6	.03	.06	.02	.05	-.44	.77													
D7	-.21	.10	-.40	.13	.26	-.20	.62												
D8	.26	-.16	.06	-.28	-.06	-.08	-.25	.69											
D9	-.19	.04	-.01	.05	-.18	.04	-.21	-.20	.85										
D10	-.36	.19	-.27	.16	.10	-.21	.00	-.16	.03	.73									
D11	-.46	.05	-.08	.30	.23	-.20	.16	-.28	-.03	.09	.63								
D12	.24	-.22	.24	-.36	-.20	.08	-.01	.06	-.15	-.58	-.18	.60							
D13	-.08	.17	-.12	-.11	.16	-.16	-.02	.05	.03	-.05	-.04	-.06	.75						
D14	-.03	-.14	.34	.03	-.28	.24	-.15	-.01	.01	-.02	.02	-.06	-.36	.38					
D15	.05	-.16	.24	-.11	-.02	.19	-.23	-.01	-.10	-.24	.03	.25	-.15	.12	.45				
D16	.25	-.09	.04	-.14	-.09	-.13	-.26	.12	.09	-.03	-.29	.20	-.06	-.10	-.08	.55			
D17	-.15	.17	-.07	.19	.02	-.08	.16	-.25	-.02	.05	.20	-.21	.04	-.03	-.12	-.40	.63		
D18	.15	-.05	.29	-.19	-.18	.06	-.19	.23	-.07	-.20	-.39	.07	-.20	.19	.09	.16	-.20	.62	
D19	.11	.10	-.11	.10	.01	.01	.34	.00	-.21	-.17	.03	.09	.02	-.15	-.10	-.22	.02	-.08	.48

Tab. A 6: Anti-image correlation matrix and measures of sample adequacy of the IPQ-R part III (Source: Own data)

	1.	2.	3.	4.	5.	6.	7.	8.	9.	10.
1. TLA		0.16	0.41*	0.12	0.09	-0.01	0.15	0.14	-0.03	0.04
2. TLC			0.46*	0.22*	-0.08	-0.19	0.47*	0.27*	0.13	0.15
3. CSQ				0.19	-0.19	-0.15	0.44*	0.16	0.11	0.13
4. PCR					0.31*	0.25*	-0.10	-0.01	0.08	-0.05
5. TCR						0.22	-0.21	0.02	0.10	0.00
6. ILC							-0.32*	-0.28*	-0.13	-0.23*
7. ERP								0.44*	0.15	0.16
8. $PSY-CA									0.47*	0.38*
9. $RFE-CA										0.30*
10. $CHA-CA										

* p<0.05

Tab. A 7: Correlation matrix of IPQ-R part II and III dimensions (Source: Own data)

A.2   Additional figures

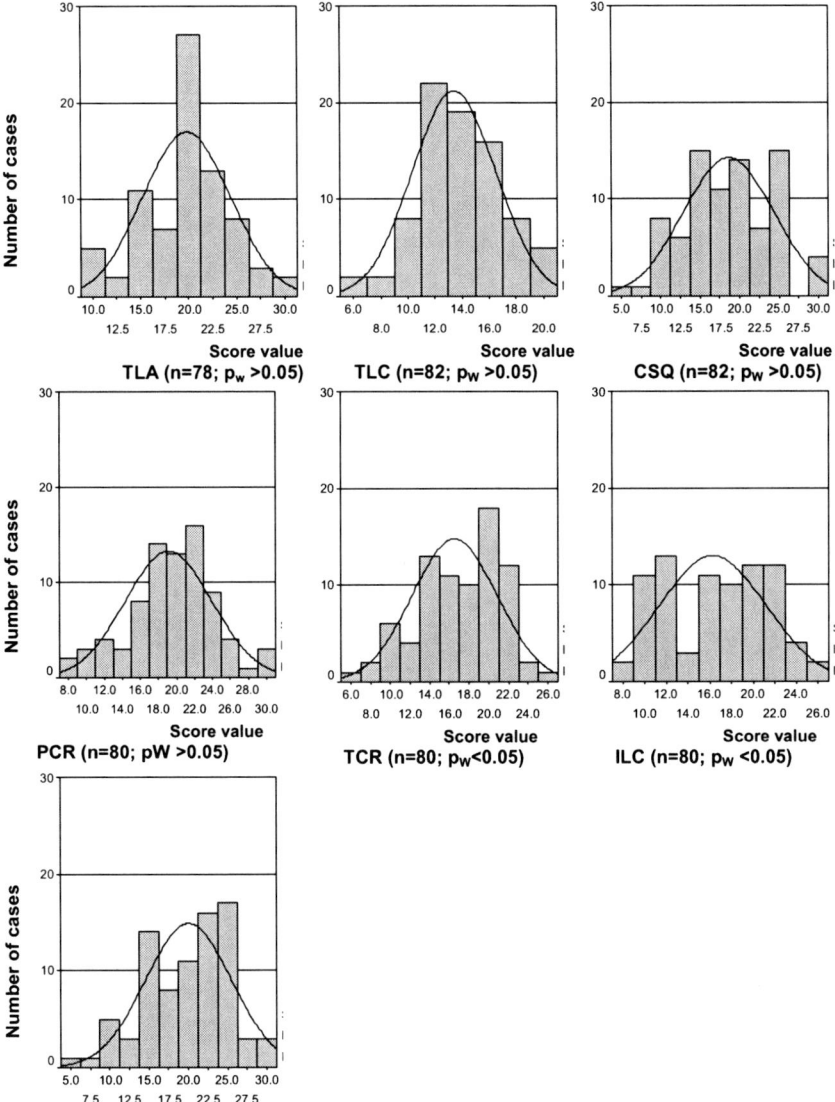

Note. P-value (p$_w$) is based on Shapiro-Wilks-test of the null hypotheses that the score distribution does not differ from a normal distribution

Fig. A 1: Distribution of the 7 IPQ-R dimensions on core beliefs (part II) over all respondents (Source: Own illustration)

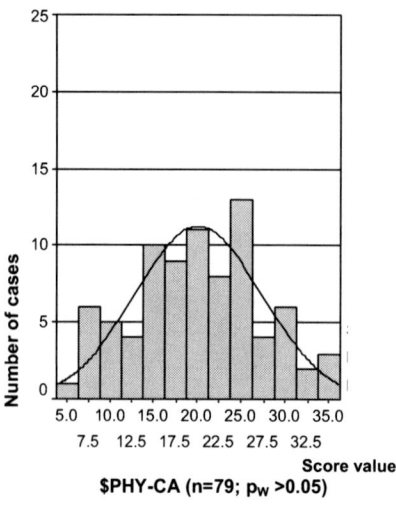

$PHY-CA (n=79; p_w >0.05)

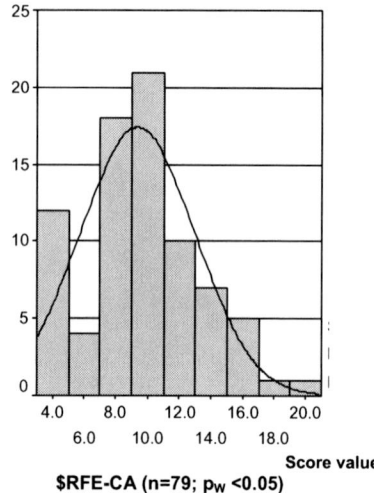

$RFE-CA (n=79; p_w <0.05)

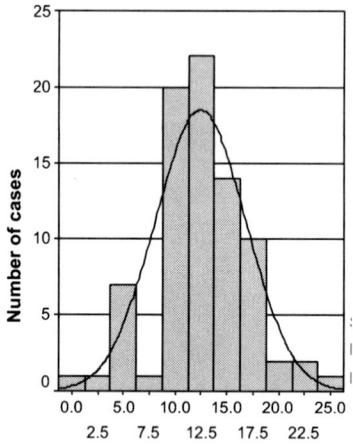

$CHA-CA (n=79; p_w >0.05)

Note. P-value (p_w) is based on Shapiro-Wilks-test of the null hypotheses that the score distribution does not differ from a normal distribution

Fig. A 2: Distribution of the 3 revised causal attributions dimension (part III)
(Source: Own illustration)

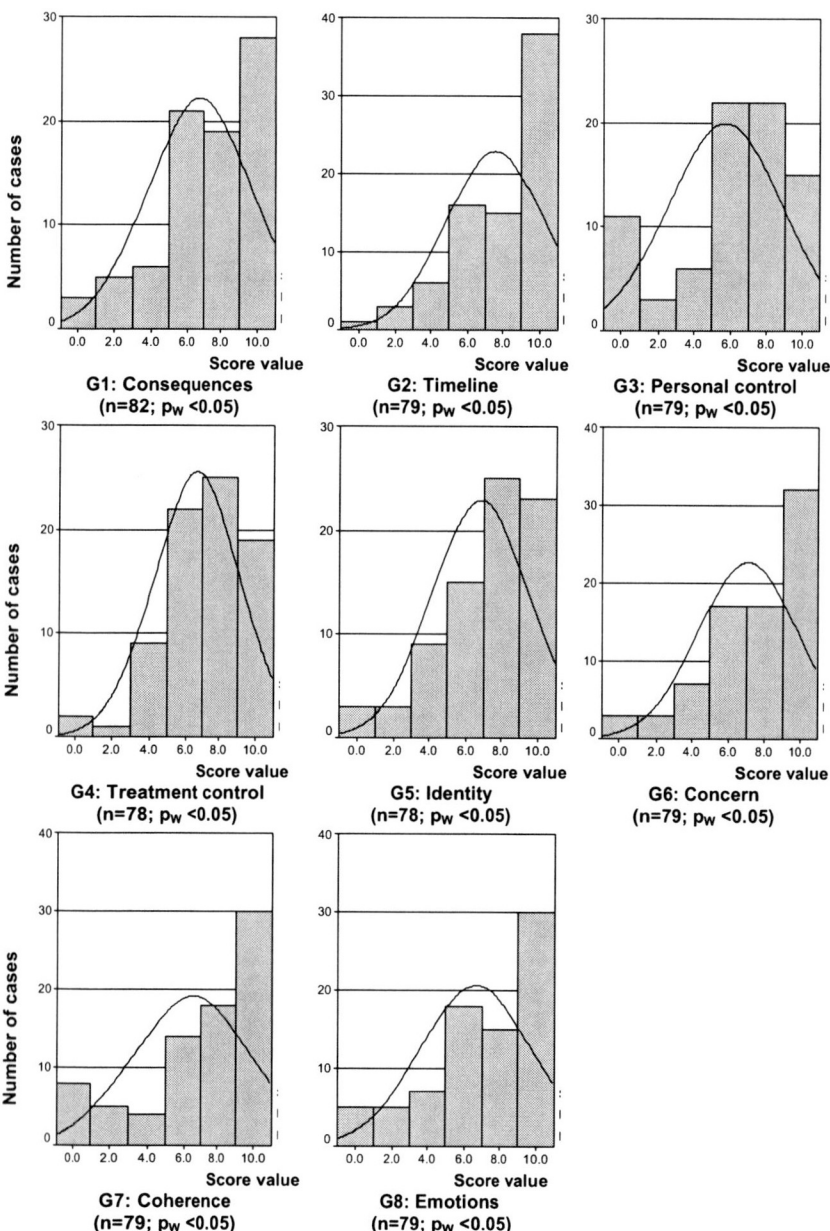

Note. P-value (pw) is based on Shapiro-Wilks-test of the null hypotheses that the score distribution does not differ from a normal distribution

Fig. A 3: Distribution of Brief IPQ items across all respondents (Source: Own data)

Appendix B: Methods of literature review

For all reviews carried out for the background part of this report, systematic literature search was done using the databases PubMed, PsycInfo, The Cochrane Library, CINHAL, and Science Citation Index for journal articles and the German and the American National Library for monographs and handbooks.

Reference lists of literature found were scanned manually for relevant sources. Where appropriate, the search strategy comprised search using Medical Subject Headings (MeSH-Terms) and search using strings in titles and abstracts. Search strings used for the different topics are listed below. They were adjusted for the requirements of each data base. Journal articles found were downloaded to a Reference Manager 11 data base (Thomson ResearchSoft 2005) and their abstracts were reviewed. Exclusion criteria are listed below next to the search strings. In general, only German and English language articles were included for review purposes. Comments and letters published in journals were excluded. Relevant articles were accessed online where possible using access over the University of Bielefeld and retrieved in printed version over the University of Bielefeld or its inter-library loan system. Hand search of journals was performed in some cases. In the following, search strings used for the different sections of this paper will be outlined:

Chapter 3.2: Review on instruments for the assessment of illness beliefs

The search string comprised the respective name of the instrument using the data bases and method outlined above.

Chapter 3.3: Review on the role of illness perceptions for coping behavior

The following search string was used: "illness AND (perception OR representation OR attitude OR belief OR conception OR cognition OR attribution) AND (adherence OR compliance OR attendance) AND (cardiac* OR heart OR hypertension OR anti-coagulation OR myocard* OR coronar*)". Search was restricted to articles published from 1990 to 2008. Only articles relevant to cardiovascular diseases were considered.

In order to compare effects reported by studies to each other, effect sizes were calculated. Instead of Cohen's d, the more complex effect size Hedge's g was used. To take into account the generally small sample sizes that were found in the studies, a special variant of Hedge's g was calculated designed to adjust for small sample sizes. This is recommended by several authors (Hedges und Olkin 1985; Cochrane Collaboration 2003). The formula used for calculation is

$$g = \frac{\bar{x}_1 - \bar{x}_2}{s_{pooled}} \left(1 - \frac{3}{4(n_1 + n_2) - 9}\right) \text{ , while } s_{pooled} = \sqrt{\frac{(n_1 - 1)s_1^2 + (n_2 - 1)s_2^2}{n_1 + n_2 - 2}}$$

In order to present summery measures for the influence of beliefs about stress and own behavior, summary $\bar{g}$'s were calculated treating effect sizes as ge-

	strongly disagree	dis-agree	neither agree nor disagree	agree	strongly agree
10. My illness has serious financial consequences	☐	☐	☐	☐	☐
11. My illness causes difficulties for those who are close to me	☐	☐	☐	☐	☐
12. There is a lot I can do to control my illness	☐	☐	☐	☐	☐
13. What I do can determine whether my illness gets better or worse	☐	☐	☐	☐	☐
14. The course of my illness depends on me	☐	☐	☐	☐	☐
15. Nothing I do will affect my illness	☐	☐	☐	☐	☐
16. I have the power to influence my illness	☐	☐	☐	☐	☐
17. My actions will have no effect on the outcome of my illness	☐	☐	☐	☐	☐
18. My illness will improve in time	☐	☐	☐	☐	☐
19. There is very little that can be done to improve my illness	☐	☐	☐	☐	☐
20. Treatment will be effective in treating my illness	☐	☐	☐	☐	☐
21. The negative effects of my illness can be prevented (avoided by my treatment)	☐	☐	☐	☐	☐
22. Treatment can control my illness	☐	☐	☐	☐	☐
23. There is nothing that can help my illness	☐	☐	☐	☐	☐
24. My illness is puzzling to me	☐	☐	☐	☐	☐
25. My illness is a mystery to me	☐	☐	☐	☐	☐
26. I don't understand my illness	☐	☐	☐	☐	☐
27. My illness doesn't make any sense to me	☐	☐	☐	☐	☐
28. I have a clear picture or understanding of my illness	☐	☐	☐	☐	☐
29. The symptoms of my illness are puzzling to me	☐	☐	☐	☐	☐
30. My symptoms come and go in circles	☐	☐	☐	☐	☐
31. My illness is very unpredictable	☐	☐	☐	☐	☐
32. I go through cycles in which my illness gets better and worse	☐	☐	☐	☐	☐
33. I get depressed when I think about my illness	☐	☐	☐	☐	☐
34. When I think about my illness I get upset	☐	☐	☐	☐	☐
35. My illness makes me feel angry	☐	☐	☐	☐	☐
36. My illness does not worry me	☐	☐	☐	☐	☐
37. My illness makes me feel anxious	☐	☐	☐	☐	☐
38. My illness makes me feel afraid	☐	☐	☐	☐	☐

We are interested to know what you think may have been the cause of your illness. Because people are very different, there is no correct or false answer to this question. We are more interested in your personal views on the factors that caused your illness rather than in what others, including doctors or your family may have said. Below a list of possible causes is given. Please indicate how much you agree or disagree with the following aspects as possible causes of your illness.

	strongly disagree	dis-agree	neither agree nor disagree	agree	strongly agree
Stress or worry	☐	☐	☐	☐	☐
Heredity – it runs in my family	☐	☐	☐	☐	☐
A germ or a virus	☐	☐	☐	☐	☐
Diet or eating habits	☐	☐	☐	☐	☐
Chance or bad luck	☐	☐	☐	☐	☐
Poor medical care in the past	☐	☐	☐	☐	☐
Pollution in the environment	☐	☐	☐	☐	☐
My own behavior	☐	☐	☐	☐	☐
My mental attitude, e.g. thinking about life negatively	☐	☐	☐	☐	☐
Family problems or worries caused my illness	☐	☐	☐	☐	☐
Overwork	☐	☐	☐	☐	☐
My emotional state, e.g. feeling down lonely, anxious, empty	☐	☐	☐	☐	☐
Aging	☐	☐	☐	☐	☐
Alcohol	☐	☐	☐	☐	☐
Smoking	☐	☐	☐	☐	☐
Accident or injury	☐	☐	☐	☐	☐
My personality	☐	☐	☐	☐	☐
Altered immunity	☐	☐	☐	☐	☐

C.2   The Brief Illness Perception Questionnaire
(Broadbent et al. 2006; also available from http://www.uib.no/ipq/)

For the following questions, please circle the number that best corresponds to your views:

How much does your illness affect your life?

         0   1 2 3 4 5 6 7 8 9 10

no affect at all   severely affects my life

How long do you think your illness will continue?

         0   1 2 3 4 5 6 7 8 9 10

 a very short time   forever

How much control do you feel you have over your illness?

        0   1 2 3 4 5 6 7 8 9 10

 absolutely no con-   extreme amount of control
trol

How much do you think your treatment can help your illness?

        0   1 2 3 4 5 6 7 8 9 10

   not at all   extremely helpful

How much do you experience symptoms from your illness?

       0   1 2 3 4 5 6 7 8 9 10

 no symptoms at all   many severe symptoms

How concerned are you about your illness?

        0   1 2 3 4 5 6 7 8 9 10

not at all concerned   extremely concerned

How well do you feel you understand your illness?

        0   1 2 3 4 5 6 7 8 9 10

don't understand at   understand very clearly
all

How much does your illness affect you emotionally? (e.g. does it make you angry, scared, upset or depressed?)

        0   1 2 3 4 5 6 7 8 9 10

  not at all affected   extremely affected emotionally
     emotionally

Please list in rank-order the three most important factors that you believe caused your illness. The most important causes for me:
1. _____
2. _____
3. _____

Appendix D: Excerpt of the research instrument

The following is a translated excerpt (section B to E) of the questionnaire applied in this study comprising the slightly modified version of the IPQ-R. The SF-12 (section A) and the PANAS (section F) are not shown.

B. Here you will find a series of symptoms that you might have experienced since the beginning of your illness. Please indicate by a cross on Yes or No, if you have experienced any of these symptoms since the beginning of your illness, and if you feel that these symptoms are related to this disease.

	I have experienced this symptom *since the beginning of my illness*		This symptom *is related to my disease*	
Pain	☐ Yes	☐ No	☐ Yes	☐ No
Sore Throat	☐ Yes	☐ No	☐ Yes	☐ No
Nausea	☐ Yes	☐ No	☐ Yes	☐ No
Breathlessness	☐ Yes	☐ No	☐ Yes	☐ No
Weight Loss	☐ Yes	☐ No	☐ Yes	☐ No
Stiff Joints	☐ Yes	☐ No	☐ Yes	☐ No
Fatigue	☐ Yes	☐ No	☐ Yes	☐ No
Sore Eyes	☐ Yes	☐ No	☐ Yes	☐ No
Wheeziness	☐ Yes	☐ No	☐ Yes	☐ No
Headaches	☐ Yes	☐ No	☐ Yes	☐ No
Upset Stomach	☐ Yes	☐ No	☐ Yes	☐ No
Sleep Difficulties	☐ Yes	☐ No	☐ Yes	☐ No
Dizziness	☐ Yes	☐ No	☐ Yes	☐ No
Loss of Strength	☐ Yes	☐ No	☐ Yes	☐ No

C. We are interested in your own personal views of how you now see your illness. Please indicate by an X how much you agree or disagree with the following statements about your illness.

	I don't think so at all	I don't think so	I am unde-cided	I think so	I absolutly think so
1. My illness will last a short time	☐	☐	☐	☐	☐
2. My illness is likely to be permanent rather than temporary	☐	☐	☐	☐	☐
3. My illness will last a long time	☐	☐	☐	☐	☐
4. This illness will pass quickly	☐	☐	☐	☐	☐
5. I expect to have this illness for the rest of my life	☐	☐	☐	☐	☐
6. My illness is a serious condition	☐	☐	☐	☐	☐
7. My illness has major consequences on my life	☐	☐	☐	☐	☐
8. My illness does not have much effect on my life	☐	☐	☐	☐	☐

	I don't think so at all	I don't think so	I am unde-cided	I think so	I absolutly think so
9. My illness strongly affects the way other see me	☐	☐	☐	☐	☐
10. My illness has serious financial consequences	☐	☐	☐	☐	☐
11. My illness causes difficulties for those who are close to me	☐	☐	☐	☐	☐
12. There is a lot I can do to control my illness	☐	☐	☐	☐	☐
13. What I do can determine whether my illness gets better or worse	☐	☐	☐	☐	☐
14. The course of my illness depends on me	☐	☐	☐	☐	☐
15. Nothing I do will affect my illness	☐	☐	☐	☐	☐
16. I have the power to influence my illness	☐	☐	☐	☐	☐
17. My actions will have no effect on the outcome of my illness	☐	☐	☐	☐	☐
18. My illness will improve in time	☐	☐	☐	☐	☐
19. There is very little that can be done to improve my illness	☐	☐	☐	☐	☐
20. Treatment will be effective in treating my ill-ness	☐	☐	☐	☐	☐
21. The negative effects of my illness can be pre-vented (avoided by my treatment)	☐	☐	☐	☐	☐
22. Treatment can control my illness	☐	☐	☐	☐	☐
23. There is nothing that can help my illness	☐	☐	☐	☐	☐
24. The symptoms of my illness are puzzling to me	☐	☐	☐	☐	☐
25. My illness is meaningless to me	☐	☐	☐	☐	☐
26. I don't understand my illness	☐	☐	☐	☐	☐
27. My illness doesn't make any sense to me	☐	☐	☐	☐	☐
28. I have a clear picture or understanding of my illness	☐	☐	☐	☐	☐
29. The symptoms of my illness change day by day	☐	☐	☐	☐	☐
30. My symptoms come and go in circles	☐	☐	☐	☐	☐
31. My illness is very unpredictable	☐	☐	☐	☐	☐
32. I go through cycles in which my illness gets bet-ter and worse	☐	☐	☐	☐	☐
33. I get depressed when I think about my illness	☐	☐	☐	☐	☐
34. When I think about my illness I get upset	☐	☐	☐	☐	☐
35. My illness makes me feel angry	☐	☐	☐	☐	☐
36. My illness does not worry me	☐	☐	☐	☐	☐
37. My illness makes me feel anxious	☐	☐	☐	☐	☐
38. My illness makes me feel afraid	☐	☐	☐	☐	☐

D. What do you think may have been the cause of your illness? Because people are very different, there is no correct or false answer to this question. Below is given a list of possible causes of his illness. Please indicate how much you think that the following aspects are possible causes of your illness.

	I don't think so at all	I don't think so	I am unde-cided	I think so	I absolutly think so
1. Stress or worry	☐	☐	☐	☐	☐
2. Heredity	☐	☐	☐	☐	☐
3. A germ or a virus	☐	☐	☐	☐	☐
4. Diet or eating habits	☐	☐	☐	☐	☐
5. Chance or bad luck	☐	☐	☐	☐	☐
6. Poor medical care in the past	☐	☐	☐	☐	☐
7. Pollution in the environment	☐	☐	☐	☐	☐
8. My own behavior	☐	☐	☐	☐	☐
9. My mental attitude, e.g. thinking about life negatively	☐	☐	☐	☐	☐
10. Family problems or worries	☐	☐	☐	☐	☐
11. Overwork	☐	☐	☐	☐	☐
12. My emotional state, e.g. feeling down lonely, anxious, empty	☐	☐	☐	☐	☐
13. Aging	☐	☐	☐	☐	☐
14. God's will					
15. Smoking or alcohol	☐	☐	☐	☐	☐
16. Accident or injury	☐	☐	☐	☐	☐
17. My personality	☐	☐	☐	☐	☐
18. Altered immunity	☐	☐	☐	☐	☐
19. Nazar	☐	☐	☐	☐	☐

E. In the table below, please list in rank-order the three most important factors that you now believe caused your illness. You may use any of the items from the box above, or you may have additional ideas of your own.

The most important causes for me:

1. ✎ _____

2. ✎ _____

3. ✎ _____

G. For the following questions, please circle the number that best corresponds to your views. Responses of the questionnaire are rated between 0 and 10. Please tick off the number that is right according to your opinion.

How much does your illness affect your life?

0 1 2 3 4 5 6 7 8 9 10

My illness does not affect my life at all

My illness does not affects my life severely

How long do you think your illness will continue?

0 1 2 3 4 5 6 7 8 9 10

My illness will last a short time

My illness will last a short time

How much control do you think you have over your illness?

0 1 2 3 4 5 6 7 8 9 10

Absolutely no control

Full control

How much do you think your treatment can help your illness?

0 1 2 3 4 5 6 7 8 9 10

My treatment cannot help me at all

My treatment can help me very much

How much do you experience symptoms from your illness?

0 1 2 3 4 5 6 7 8 9 10

I experience no symptoms at all

I experience many severe symptoms

How concerned are you about your illness?

0 1 2 3 4 5 6 7 8 9 10

I am not concerned at all

I am extremely concerned

How well do you feel you understand your illness?

0 1 2 3 4 5 6 7 8 9 10

I do not understand my illness at all

I understand my illness very much/good

How much does your illness affect you emotionally? *(e.g. does it make you angry, scared, upset or depressed?)*

0 1 2 3 4 5 6 7 8 9 10

My illness does not affected emotionally at all

My illness does not affected emotionally at all

Appendix E: Structured topic guide (Turkish/English)

Sonunda anket formu üzeri fikirlerinizi almak istiyoruz. Finally, we would like to known your opinion about the questionnaire.

1.**Anket üzerine izleniminiz nasıl?** *What impression do you have of the questionnaire?*

2.**Anlamadığınız veya iki anlamlı olan kelimeler veya cümleler var mıydı?** *Are there any words or phrases that perhaps are ambiguous or that you do not understand?*

3.**Kullanılan dili ve tarzı nasıl buldunuz?** *What do you think about the language and style used?*

4.**Kolaylıkla anlaşılıyor mu yoksa çok bilimsel ve resmimi?** *Is the questionnaire easy to understand or too formal and scientific?*

5.**Örnek olarak tekliferiniz var mı?** *Do you have any suggestions for improvement?*

Index

Challenges in Public Health

Im Zeitalter der Globalisierung lässt sich *Public Health* nicht mehr allein innerhalb von nationalen Grenzen betreiben: Pandemien, abnehmende Trinkwasservorräte und steigender Tabakkonsum sind nur einige Beispiele für eine Vielzahl von neuen Herausforderungen, die einen weiter reichenden, internationalen Blick erfordern. Zusätzlich trägt eine einseitig an Wirtschaftsinteressen orientierte Globalisierung zu der weltweit zunehmenden gesundheitlichen Ungleichheit bei. Die Globalisierung eröffnet andererseits aber neue Wege, auch über Staatsgrenzen und große Entfernungen hinweg Wissen und Erfahrungen auszutauschen und gemeinschaftlich zu handeln. Kernpunkte für *Public Health* sind dabei die international vergleichende Analyse von Gesundheitsproblemen und möglichen Lösungsansätzen sowie die wissenschaftlich basierte und gerechte Ausgestaltung von Gesundheitssystemen. Hierzu möchte die Buchreihe *Challenges in Public Health* einen Beitrag leisten.

In times of globalisation, Public Health can no longer be practiced within national borders alone. Pandemics, diminishing drinking water supplies and increasing tobacco consumption are examples of the many new challenges that require a cross-border, international approach. In addition, a globalisation that is narrowly focused on economic interests contributes to growing health inequalities worldwide. At the same time, globalisation offers new opportunities to exchange knowledge and experiences and to collaborate across national borders. Key issues for Public Health are an international comparison of health problems and of possible strategies to solve them, as well as an evidence-based and equitable development of health systems. The book series *Challenges in Public Health* aims to contribute to this endeavour.

Medizin in Entwicklungsländern

Herausgegeben von Prof. Hans Jochen Diesfeld

Band 1 Wolfgang Bichmann: Die Problematik der Gesundheitsplanung in Entwicklungsländern. Ein Beitrag zur Geschichte, der Situation und den Perspektiven der Planung des nationalen Gesundheitswesens in den > Least Developed Countries < Afrikas. 1979.

Band 2 Jens Herrmann: Ambition and Reality - Planning for Health and Basic Health Services in the Yemen Arab Republic. 1979.

Band 3 J.M. Pönninghaus: The Cost Benefit of Measles Immunisation. A Study from Southern Zambia. 1979.

Band 4 Hilde Wander (Hrsg.): Bedingungen und Möglichkeiten der Integrierung bevölkerungspolitischer Programme in die nationale und die internationale Entwicklungspolitik. 1980.

Band 5 M. Heidegger/H.J. Diesfeld/A. Selheim: Demographische und soziale Wirkungen von Familienplanung. 1980.

Band 6 H.J. Diesfeld (Hrsg.): Importierte Krankheiten und ärztliche Untersuchungen vor und nach Tropenaufenthalt. Kongreßbericht über die X. Tagung der Deutschen Tropenmedizinischen Gesellschaft vom 22.-24. März 1979 in Heidelberg. 1980.

Band 7 Alexander Boroffka: Benedict Nta Tanka's Commentary and Dramatized Ideas on "Disease and Witchcraft in our Society". A Schreber Case from Cameroon Annotated Autobiographical Notes by an African on his Mental Illness. 1980.

Band 8 Hartmut Brandt: Work Capacity Restraints in Tropical Agricultural Development. 1980.

Band 9 nicht erschienen

Band 10 Tilman Nitzschke / Donata von Lüttwitz: Annehmbarkeit präventiver und promotiver Maßnahmen eines Health Centre für die Bevölkerung. Dargestellt am Beispiel der ländlichen Gesundheitsversorgung der Vereinigten Republik Kamerun. 1981.

Band 11 H.J. Diesfeld (Ed.): Health Research in Developing Countries. Proceedings of the Joint Meeting of the Belgische Vereniging voor Tropische Geneeskunde, Societé Belge de Medecine Tropicale, the Nederlandse Vereniging voor Tropische Geneeskunde and the Deutsche Tropenmedizinische Gesellschaft. 1982.

Band 12 Axel Kroeger/Francoise Barbira-Freedman: Cultural Change and Health: The Case of Southamerican Rainforest Indians. With special reference to the Shuar/Achuar of Ecuador. 1982.

Band 13 Dorothea Sich: Mutterschaft und Geburt im Kulturwandel. Ein Beitrag zur transkulturellen Gesundheitsforschung aus Korea. 1982.

Band 14 Uwe K. Brinkmann: Onchozerkose in Westafrika. 1982.

Band 15 Peter Oberender/Hans Jochen Diesfeld/Wolfgang Gitter (Hrsg.): Health and Development in Africa. International, Interdisciplinary Symposium, 2-4 June 1982, University of Bayreuth. 1983.

Band 16 Josef Boch (Hrsg.): Tropenmedizin, Parasitologie, Trypanosomiasis, Malaria, Bilharziose, Onchozerkose, Importierte Virusinfektionen, Lepra, Intermediate Technology, Zecken und durch sie übertragene Krankheiten, Immundiagnostik. 1984.

Band 17 Abdin Hamid Shaddad: Anforderungen an Gesundheitseinrichtungen der Basisversorgung im Sudan. Ein Beitrag zur Gesundheitsversorgung und zu baulichen Maßnahmen für die Gesundheitseinrichtungen unter besonderer Berücksichtigung der vorhandenen Ressourcen, der sozialen Verhältnisse und der klimatischen Bedingungen. 1984.

Band 18 Gerhard Heller: Krankheitskonzepte und Krankheitssymptome. Eine empirische Untersuchung bei den Tamang von Cautara/Nepal zur Frage der kulturspezifischen Prägung von Krankheitserleben. 1985.

Band 19 Hans-Jochen Diesfeld / Sigrid Wolter (Hrsg.): Medizin in Entwicklungsländern. Handbuch zur praxisorientierten Vorbereitung für medizinische Entwicklungshelfer. 5. neubearbeitete Auflage. 1989.

Band 20 Verena Kücholl: Soziokulturelle Wege des Heilens. Eine ethnomedizinische Analyse und Interpretation des Samkhya und der Heiltradition der Navajo. 1985.

Band 21 Frank-Peter Schelp (Ed.): Health Problems in Asia and in the Federal Republic of Germany. How to solve them? Proceedings of a seminar on "Techniques and Problems of Intervention Trials in Developing and Developed Countries". 1985.

Band 22 Rolf Heinmüller, Winfried Kern: Primäre Gesundheitsversorgung im südwestlichen Sudan. Eine Feldforschung bei den südsudanesischen Azande zur Evaluierung der Einflüsse des 'Primary Health Care'-Programms auf gesundheitliche Lage und allgemeine Lebensbedingungen. Detailed English Summary. 1987.

Band 23 Andreas Hahold/Axel Kroeger: Krankheitsbewältigung im Andenhochland Perus. Ergebnisse einer Bevölkerungsbefragung. 1986.

Band 24 Georg Kamm / Peter Witton / Hatibu Lweno: Anaesthesia Notebook for Medical Auxilaries. With special Reference to Anaesthesia Practice in Developing Countries. 1989.

Band 25 Alice S. Kuhn: Heiler und ihre Patienten auf dem Dach der Welt. Ladakh aus ethnomedizinischer Sicht. 1988.

Band 26 Wolfgang Bichmann: Community Involvement in Nepal's Health System. A case study of district health services management and the Community Health Leader scheme in Kaski district. 1989.

Band 27 M. Luisa Vázquez / Renate Lipowsky / Axel Kroeger: Malaria und kutane Leishmaniase in Kolumbien. Vorkommen, Volkskonzepte und traditionelle Behandlungsformen. 1989.

Band 28 Heinrich Berg / Axel Kroeger / Carmen Perez-Samaniego / Fernando Malo: Kranke Menschen – krankes Gesundheitswesen? Eine epidemiologische Untersuchung in Nord-Mexiko. 1989.

Band 29 Emmie Ho-Tsui / Margit Urhahn: Medizin und Gesundheitsforschung in Entwicklungsländern. Bibliographie des Instituts für Tropenhygiene 1984-1988. 1991.

Band 30 Thomas Lux: Gespräche mit afrikanischen Krankenpflegern und Heilern. Bilder von Krankheit im Mikrokosmos von Malanville(Benin), 1991.

Band 31 Christopher Knauth: Arzneimittelgebrauch armer Bevölkerungsschichten in städtischen Elendsvierteln Perus. Möglichkeiten und Grenzen der Gesundheitserziehung zum rationalen Arzneimittelgebrauch. 1991.

Band 32 Erhard Hinz: Geomedizinische und biogeographische Aspekte der Krankheitsverbreitung und Gesundheitsversorgung in Industrie- und Entwicklungsländern. 1991.

Band 33 Klaus Hoffmann: Psychiatrie in Afrika. Eine Einführung für Entwicklungshelfer. 1992.

Band 34 Dorothea Sich / Hans Jochen Diesfeld / Angelika Deigner / Monika Habermann (Hrsg.): Medizin und Kultur. Eine Propädeutik für Studierende der Medizin und der Ethnologie mit 4 Seminaren in Kulturvergleichender Medizinischer Anthropologie (KMA). 1993. 2., unveränd. Aufl. 1995.

Band 35 Annette Wiemann-Michaels: Die verhexte Speise. Eine ethnopsychosomatische Studie über das Depressive Syndrom in Nepal. 1994.

Band 36 Christine Loytved: Hebammen in Ozeanien zwischen traditioneller und westlicher Medizin. Weiterbildung traditioneller Hebammen in Westsamoa und Tonga. 1994.

Band 37 Andrea Materlik: Medizinisch-anthropologische Aspekte von Lepra im Amazonas und ihre Bedeutung für die Gesundheitserziehung. 1994.

Band 38 Oliver Razum: Improving Service Quality through Action Research, as applied in the Expanded Programme on Immunization (EPI). 1994.

Band 39 Ulrich Schramm: Einflußfaktoren auf die Akzeptanz von baulichen Anlagen der ländlichen Gesundheitseinheiten in Ägypten. Fallstudie am Beispiel der staatlichen Einheit in Zebeda unter Verwendung der Post-Occupancy Evaluation. 1995.

Band 40 Rainer Sauerborn / Adrien Nougtara / Hans Jochen Diesfeld (Eds.): Recherche sur les systèmes de santé: Le cas de la zone médicale de Solenzo, Burkina Faso. Auteurs: Rainer Sauerborn, Adrien Nougtara, Hans Jochen Diesfeld, Gaston Sorgho, Joseph Bidiga, Lougousse Tiébélessé, Eric Latimer, Roberto Sallier de La Tour, Uwe Brinkmann, Don Shepard. 1995.

Band 41 Rainer Sauerborn / Adrien Nougtara / Hans Jochen Diesfeld (Eds.): Les Côuts Economiques de la Maladie pour les Ménages au Milieu Rural du Burkina Faso. Avec des contributions de Rainer Sauerborn, Adrien Nougtara, Maurice Hien, Issouf Ibrango, Matthias Borchert, Justus Benzler, Eberhard Koob, Hans Jochen Diesfeld. 1996.

Band 42 Erhard Hinz: Helminthiasen des Menschen in Thailand. 1996.

Band 43 Matthias Perleth: Historical Aspects of American Trypanosomiasis (Chagas' Disease). 1997.

Band 44 Christiane Fischer: Über die Effektivität der Dorfgesundheitsarbeiterinnen innerhalb der Nichtregierungsorganisation ACCORD in Tamil Nadu/Südindien. Aktionsforschung im Rahmen der Gesundheitssystemforschung. 1998.

Band 45 Maureen Dar lang: Assessment of antenatal and obstetric care services in a rural district of Nepal. 1999.

Band 46 Julia Katzan: sòi mendan – Die Sache mit dem Wasser... Eine medizinethnologische Untersuchung zum Zusammenhang von Wasser und Krankheit aus indigener Sicht. 2001.

Band 47 Catharina Will: Malaria-Selbstmedikation mit Chloroquin in einem hyperendemischen Gebiet (Mali). 2001.

Band 48 Ansgar Gerhardus: Entscheidungsprozesse im Gesundheitssektor. Der Beitrag der Theorie der politischen Ökonomie. 2001.

Band 49 Sylvie Schuster: Der Schwangerschaftsabbruch im Grasland Kameruns. Medizin, Kultur und Praxis. 2004.

Band 50 Sascha Klotzbücher: Das ländliche Gesundheitswesen der VR China. Strukturen – Akteure – Dynamik. 2006.

Challenges in Public Health

Editor: Prof. Dr. Oliver Razum

Band 51 Ulrich Ronellenfitsch: Cardiovascular Mortality among Ethnic German Immigrants from the Former Soviet Union. 2007.

Band 52 Manuela De Allegri: To Enrol or not to Enrol in Community Health Insurance. Case Study from Burkina Faso. 2007.

Band 53 Catherine Kyobutungi: Ethnic German Immigrants from the Former Soviet Union: Mortality from External Causes and Cancers. 2008.

Band 54 Maren Bredehorst: Information Systems for the Rehabilitation of Landmine Survivors. 2007.

Band 55 Sven Voigtländer / Gabriele Berg-Beckhoff / Oliver Razum: Gesundheitliche Ungleichheit. Der Beitrag kontextueller Merkmale. 2008.

Band 56 Oliver Razum / Jürgen Breckenkamp / Pitt Reitmaier (Hrsg.): Kindergesundheit in Entwicklungsländern. 2008.

Band 57 Steffen Fleßa: Costing of Health Care Services in Developing Countries. A Prerequisite for Affordability, Sustainability and Efficiency. 2009.

Band 58 Patrick Brzoska / Oliver Razum: Validity Issues in Quantitative Migrant Health Research. The Example of Illness Perceptions. 2010.

www.peterlang.de

Peter Lang · Internationaler Verlag der Wissenschaften

Erhabor S. Idemudia / Klaus Boehnke

I'm an Alien in Deutschland
A Quantitative Mental Health Case Study of African Immigrants in Germany
With an Epilogue by John W. Berry

Frankfurt am Main, Berlin, Bern, Bruxelles, New York, Oxford, Wien, 2010.
130 pp., 1 fig., num tab.
ISBN 978-3-631-59975-4 · pb. € 22,80*

The book presents a study of – legal, illegal, and incarcerated – African immigrants in Germany. Participants responded to a selection of scales from the Minnesota Multiphasic Personality Inventory (MMPI-2), the Portrait Value Questionnaire (PVQ) by Schwartz, and a measure of acculturative stress. Acculturative stress and German racism emerged as strong predictors of poor mental health, with problems becoming worse over the years of stay in Germany. Particularly among 'economic refugees' a precarious job situation and family fragmentation added grossly to acculturative stress. As John W. Berry, the nestor of acculturation research puts it in his epilogue: "What can only help is an increase in basic hospitality: Making African immigrants welcome in their new home is needed, not a bulwark Europe."

Content: Legal, illegal, and incarcerated African immigrants in Germany · Mental health · Acculturative stress · Value preferences · Family fragmentation · German racism · Higher acculturative stress with increasing duration of stay in Germany · Structural equation modeling · 'Economic refugees' · Precarious job situation · Daily hassles

Frankfurt am Main · Berlin · Bern · Bruxelles · New York · Oxford · Wien
Distribution: Verlag Peter Lang AG
Moosstr. 1, CH-2542 Pieterlen
Telefax 00 41 (0) 32 / 376 17 27

*The €-price includes German tax rate
Prices are subject to change without notice

Homepage http://www.peterlang.de